**Mental Health Policy and
Service Guidance Package**

MENTAL HEALTH POLICY, PLANS AND PROGRAMMES

(updated version)

World Health Organization

WHO Library Cataloguing-in-Publication Data

Mental health policy, plans and programmes - Rev. ed.
(Mental health policy and service guidance package)

1. Mental health
2. Mental health services
organization and administration
3. Public policy
4. National health programmes
organization and administration
5. Health plan implementation
6. Health planning guidelines   I. World Health Organization   II. Series.

ISBN 92 4 154646 8
(NLM classification: WM 30)

Technical information concerning this publication can be obtained from:
Dr Michelle Funk
Mental Health Policy and Service Development Team
Department of Mental Health and Substance Abuse
Noncommunicable Diseases and Mental Health Cluster
World Health Organization
CH-1211, Geneva 27
Switzerland
Tel: +41 22 791 3855
Fax: +41 22 791 4160
E-mail: funkm@who.int

© World Health Organization 2005

Printed in China

Acknowledgements

The Mental Health Policy and Service Guidance Package was produced under the direction of Dr Michelle Funk, Coordinator, Mental Health Policy and Service Development, and supervised by Dr Benedetto Saraceno, Director, Department of Mental Health and Substance Abuse, World Health Organization.

The World Health Organization gratefully thanks Dr Alberto Minoletti, Ministry of Health, Chile, who prepared this module.

Editorial and technical coordination group:

Dr Michelle Funk, World Health Organization, Headquarters (WHO/HQ), Ms Natalie Drew, (WHO/HQ), Dr JoAnne Epping-Jordan, (WHO/HQ), Mrs Margaret Grigg (WHO/HQ), Professor Alan J. Flisher, University of Cape Town, Observatory, Republic of South Africa, Professor Melvyn Freeman, Human Sciences Research Council, Pretoria, South Africa, Dr Howard Goldman, National Association of State Mental Health Program Directors Research Institute and University of Maryland School of Medicine, USA, Dr Itzhak Levav, Mental Health Services, Ministry of Health, Jerusalem, Israel and Dr Benedetto Saraceno, (WHO/HQ).

Dr Crick Lund, University of Cape Town, Observatory, Republic of South Africa finalized the technical editing of this module.

Technical assistance:

Dr Jose Bertolote, World Health Organization, Headquarters (WHO/HQ), Dr José Miguel Caldas de Almeida, WHO Regional Office for the Americas (AMRO), Dr Vijay Chandra, WHO Regional Office for South-East Asia (SEARO), Dr Custodia Mandlhate, WR/ Namibia, Dr Claudio Miranda (AMRO), Dr Ahmed Mohit, WHO Regional Office for the Eastern Mediterranean, Dr Wolfgang Rutz, WHO Regional Office for Europe (EURO), Dr WANG Xiandong, WHO Regional Office for the Western Pacific, (WRPO), Dr Derek Yach (WHO/HQ) and staff of the WHO Evidence and Information for Policy Cluster (WHO/HQ).

Administrative and secretarial support:

Ms Adeline Loo (WHO/HQ), Mrs Anne Yamada (WHO/HQ) and Mrs Razia Yaseen (WHO/HQ).

Layout and graphic design: 2S) graphicdesign
Editor: Walter Ryder

WHO also gratefully thanks the following people for their expert opinion and technical input to this module:

Dr Adel Hamid Afana	Director, Training and Education Department Gaza Community Mental Health Programme
Dr Bassam Al Ashhab	Ministry of Health, Palestinian Authority, West Bank
Mrs Ella Amir	Ami Québec, Canada
Dr Julio Arboleda-Florez	Department of Psychiatry, Queen's University, Kingston, Ontario, Canada
Ms Jeannine Auger	Ministry of Health and Social Services, Québec, Canada
Dr Florence Baingana	World Bank, Washington DC, USA
Mrs Louise Blanchette	University of Montreal Certificate Programme in Mental Health, Montreal, Canada
Dr Susan Blyth	University of Cape Town, Cape Town, South Africa
Dr Thomas Bornemann	Director, Mental Health, The Carter Centre Mental Health Program, Altanta, USA
Ms Nancy Breitenbach	Inclusion International, Ferney-Voltaire, France
Dr Anh Thu Bui	Ministry of Health, Koror, Republic of Palau
Dr Sylvia Caras	People Who Organization, Santa Cruz, California, USA
Dr Claudina Cayetano	Ministry of Health, Belmopan, Belize
Dr CHANG Chueh	Taipei, Taiwan, China
Professor YAN Fang Chen	Shandong Mental Health Centre, Jinan People's Republic of China
Dr Chantharavdy Choulamany	Mahosot General Hospital, Vientiane, Lao People's Democratic Republic
Dr Ellen Corin	Douglas Hospital Research Centre, Quebec, Canada
Dr Jim Crowe	President, World Fellowship for Schizophrenia and Allied Disorders, Dunedin, New Zealand
Dr Araba Sefa Dedeh	University of Ghana Medical School, Accra, Ghana
Dr Nimesh Desai	Professor of Psychiatry and Medical Superintendent, Institute of Human Behaviour and Allied Sciences, India
Dr M. Parameshvara Deva	Department of Psychiatry, Perak College of Medicine, Ipoh, Perak, Malaysia
Professor Saida Douki	President, Société Tunisienne de Psychiatrie, Tunis, Tunisia
Professor Ahmed Abou El-Azayem	Past President, World Federation for Mental Health, Cairo, Egypt
Dr Abra Fransch	WONCA, Harare, Zimbabwe
Dr Gregory Fricchione	Carter Center, Atlanta, USA
Dr Michael Friedman	Nathan S. Kline Institute for Psychiatric Research, Orangeburg, NY, USA
Mrs Diane Froggatt	Executive Director, World Fellowship for Schizophrenia and Allied Disorders, Toronto, Ontario, Canada
Mr Gary Furlong	Metro Local Community Health Centre, Montreal, Canada
Dr Vijay Ganju	National Association of State Mental Health Program Directors Research Institute, Alexandria, VA, USA
Mrs Reine Gobeil	Douglas Hospital, Quebec, Canada
Dr Nacanieli Goneyali	Ministry of Health, Suva, Fiji
Dr Gaston Harnois	Douglas Hospital Research Centre, WHO Collaborating Centre, Quebec, Canada
Mr Gary Haugland	Nathan S. Kline Institute for Psychiatric Research, Orangeburg, NY, USA
Dr HE Yanling	Consultant, Ministry of Health, Beijing, People's Republic of China

Professor Helen Herrman	Department of Psychiatry, University of Melbourne, Australia
Mrs Karen Hetherington	WHO/PAHO Collaborating Centre, Canada
Professor Frederick Hickling	Section of Psychiatry, University of West Indies, Kingston, Jamaica
Dr Kim Hopper	Nathan S. Kline Institute for Psychiatric Research, Orangeburg, NY, USA
Dr HWANG Tae-Yeon	Director, Department of Psychiatric Rehabilitation and Community Psychiatry, Yongin City, Republic of Korea
Dr Aleksandar Janca	University of Western Australia, Perth, Australia
Dr Dale L. Johnson	World Fellowship for Schizophrenia and Allied Disorders, Taos, NM, USA
Dr Kristine Jones	Nathan S. Kline Institute for Psychiatric Research, Orangeburg, NY, USA
Dr David Musau Kiima	Director, Department of Mental Health, Ministry of Health, Nairobi, Kenya
Mr Todd Krieble	Ministry of Health, Wellington, New Zealand
Mr John P. Kummer	Equilibrium, Unteraegeri, Switzerland
Professor Lourdes Ladrido-Ignacio	Department of Psychiatry and Behavioural Medicine, College of Medicine and Philippine General Hospital, Manila, Philippines
Dr Pirkko Lahti	Secretary-General/Chief Executive Officer, World Federation for Mental Health, and Executive Director, Finnish Association for Mental Health, Helsinki, Finland
Mr Eero Lahtinen	Ministry of Social Affairs and Health, Helsinki, Finland
Dr Eugene M. Laska	Nathan S. Kline Institute for Psychiatric Research, Orangeburg, NY, USA
Dr Eric Latimer	Douglas Hospital Research Centre, Quebec, Canada
Dr Ian Lockhart	University of Cape Town, Observatory, Republic of South Africa
Dr Marcelino López	Research and Evaluation, Andalusian Foundation for Social Integration of the Mentally Ill, Seville, Spain
Ms Annabel Lyman	Behavioural Health Division, Ministry of Health, Koror, Republic of Palau
Dr MA Hong	Consultant, Ministry of Health, Beijing, People's Republic of China
Dr George Mahy	University of the West Indies, St Michael, Barbados
Dr Joseph Mbatia	Ministry of Health, Dar es Salaam, Tanzania
Dr Céline Mercier	Douglas Hospital Research Centre, Quebec, Canada
Dr Leen Meulenbergs	Belgian Inter-University Centre for Research and Action, Health and Psychobiological and Psychosocial Factors, Brussels, Belgium
Dr Harry I. Minas	Centre for International Mental Health and Transcultural Psychiatry, St. Vincent's Hospital, Fitzroy, Victoria, Australia
Dr Alberto Minoletti	Ministry of Health, Santiago de Chile, Chile
Dr Paula Mogne	Ministry of Health, Mozambique
Dr Paul Morgan	SANE, South Melbourne, Victoria, Australia
Dr Driss Moussaoui	Université psychiatrique, Casablanca, Morocco
Dr Matt Muijen	The Sainsbury Centre for Mental Health, London, United Kingdom
Dr Carmine Munizza	Centro Studi e Ricerca in Psichiatria, Turin, Italy
Dr Shisram Narayan	St Giles Hospital, Suva, Fiji
Dr Sheila Ndyanabangi	Ministry of Health, Kampala, Uganda
Dr Grayson Norquist	National Institute of Mental Health, Bethesda, MD, USA

Dr Frank Njenga	Chairman of Kenya Psychiatrists' Association, Nairobi, Kenya
Dr Angela Ofori-Atta	Clinical Psychology Unit, University of Ghana Medical School, Korle-Bu, Ghana
Professor Mehdi Paes	Arrazi University Psychiatric Hospital, Sale, Morocco
Dr Rampersad Parasram	Ministry of Health, Port of Spain, Trinidad and Tobago
Dr Vikram Patel	Sangath Centre, Goa, India
Dr Dixianne Penney	Nathan S. Kline Institute for Psychiatric Research, Orangeburg, NY, USA
Dr Yogan Pillay	Equity Project, Pretoria, Republic of South Africa
Dr Michal Pohanka	Ministry of Health, Czech Republic
Dr Laura L. Post	Mariana Psychiatric Services, Saipan, USA
Dr Prema Ramachandran	Planning Commission, New Delhi, India
Dr Helmut Remschmidt	Department of Child and Adolescent Psychiatry, Marburg, Germany
Professor Brian Robertson	Department of Psychiatry, University of Cape Town, Republic of South Africa
Dr Julieta Rodriguez Rojas	Integrar a la Adolescencia, Costa Rica
Dr Agnes E. Rupp	Chief, Mental Health Economics Research Program, NIMH/NIH, USA
Dr Ayesh M. Sammour	Ministry of Health, Palestinian Authority, Gaza
Dr Aive Sarjas	Department of Social Welfare, Tallinn, Estonia
Dr Radha Shankar	AASHA (Hope), Chennai, India
Dr Carole Siegel	Nathan S. Kline Institute for Psychiatric Research, Orangeburg, NY, USA
Professor Michele Tansella	Department of Medicine and Public Health, University of Verona, Italy
Ms Mrinali Thalgodapitiya	Executive Director, NEST, Hendala, Watala, Gampaha District, Sri Lanka
Dr Graham Thornicroft	Director, PRISM, The Maudsley Institute of Psychiatry, London, United Kingdom
Dr Giuseppe Tibaldi	Centro Studi e Ricerca in Psichiatria, Turin, Italy
Ms Clare Townsend	Department of Psychiatry, University of Queensland, Toowing Qld, Australia
Dr Gombodorjiin Tsetsegdary	Ministry of Health and Social Welfare, Mongolia
Dr Bogdana Tudorache	President, Romanian League for Mental Health, Bucharest, Romania
Ms Judy Turner-Crowson	Former Chair, World Association for Psychosocial Rehabilitation, WAPR Advocacy Committee, Hamburg, Germany
Mrs Pascale Van den Heede	Mental Health Europe, Brussels, Belgium
Ms Marianna Várfalvi-Bognarne	Ministry of Health, Hungary
Dr Uldis Veits	Riga Municipal Health Commission, Riga, Latvia
Mr Luc Vigneault	Association des Groupes de Défense des Droits en Santé Mentale du Québec, Canada
Dr WANG Liwei	Consultant, Ministry of Health, Beijing, People's Republic of China
Dr Erica Wheeler	Ornex, France
Professor Harvey Whiteford	Department of Psychiatry, University of Queensland, Toowing Qld, Australia
Dr Ray G. Xerri	Department of Health, Floriana, Malta
Dr XIE Bin	Consultant, Ministry of Health, Beijing, People's Republic of China
Dr YU Xin	Consultant, Ministry of Health, Beijing, People's Republic of China

Professor SHEN Yucun	Institute of Mental Health, Beijing Medical University, People's Republic of China
Dr Taintor Zebulon	President, WAPR, Department of Psychiatry, New York University Medical Center, New York, USA

WHO also wishes to acknowledge the generous financial support of the Governments of Australia, Finland, Italy, the Netherlands, New Zealand, and Norway.

Table of Contents

"A mental health policy and plan is essential to coordinate all services and activities related to mental health. Without adequate policies and plans, mental disorders are likely to be treated in an inefficient and fragmented manner."

This module is part of the WHO Mental Health Policy and Service guidance package, which provides practical information to assist countries to improve the mental health of their populations.

What is the purpose of the guidance package?

The purpose of the guidance package is to assist policy-makers and planners to:

- develop policies and comprehensive strategies for improving the mental health of populations;

- use existing resources to achieve the greatest possible benefits;

- provide effective services to those in need;

- assist the reintegration of persons with mental disorders into all aspects of community life, thus improving their overall quality of life.

What is in the package?

The package consists of a series of interrelated user-friendly modules that are designed to address the wide variety of needs and priorities in policy development and service planning. The topic of each module represents a core aspect of mental health. The starting point is the module entitled The Mental Health Context, which outlines the global context of mental health and summarizes the content of all the modules. This module should give readers an understanding of the global context of mental health, and should enable them to select specific modules that will be useful to them in their own situations. Mental Health Policy, Plans and Programmes is a central module, providing detailed information about the process of developing policy and implementing it through plans and programmes. Following a reading of this module, countries may wish to focus on specific aspects of mental health covered in other modules.

The guidance package includes the following modules:

> The Mental Health Context
> Mental Health Policy, Plans and Programmes
> Mental Health Financing
> Mental Health Legislation and Human Rights
> Advocacy for Mental Health
> Organization of Services for Mental Health
> Quality Improvement for Mental Health
> Planning and Budgeting to Deliver Services for Mental Health

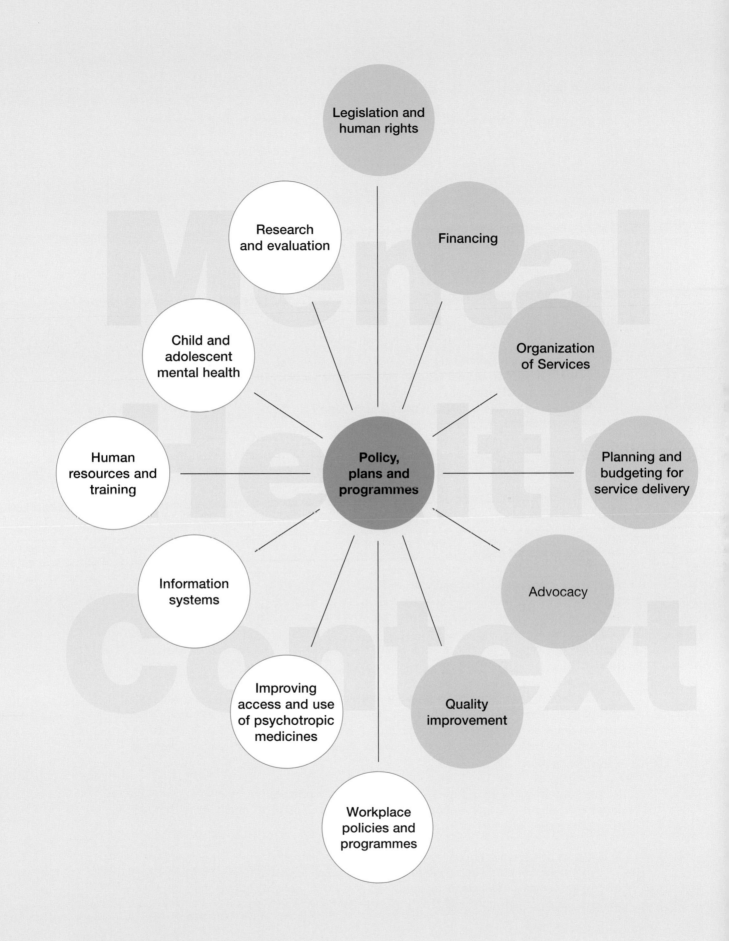

Legislation and human rights

Financing

Research and evaluation

Organization of Services

Child and adolescent mental health

Human resources and training

Policy, plans and programmes

Planning and budgeting for service delivery

Information systems

Advocacy

Improving access and use of psychotropic medicines

Quality improvement

Workplace policies and programmes

● still to be developed

The following modules are not yet available but will be included in the final guidance package:

> Improving Access and Use of Psychotropic Medicines
> Mental Health Information Systems
> Human Resources and Training for Mental Health
> Child and Adolescent Mental Health
> Research and Evaluation of Mental Health Policy and Services
> Workplace Mental Health Policies and Programmes

Who is the guidance package for?

The modules will be of interest to:

- policy-makers and health planners;
- government departments at federal, state/regional and local levels;
- mental health professionals;
- groups representing people with mental disorders;
- representatives or associations of families and carers
  of people with mental disorders;
- advocacy organizations representing the interests of people with mental
  disorders and their relatives and families;
- nongovernmental organizations involved or interested in the provision
  of mental health services.

How to use the modules

- They can be used **individually or as a package**. They are cross-referenced with each other for ease of use. Countries may wish to go through each of the modules systematically or may use a specific module when the emphasis is on a particular area of mental health. For example, countries wishing to address mental health legislation may find the module entitled Mental Health Legislation and Human Rights useful for this purpose.

- They can be used as a **training package** for mental health policy-makers, planners and others involved in organizing, delivering and funding mental health services. They can be used as educational materials in university or college courses. Professional organizations may choose to use the package as an aid to training for persons working in mental health.

- They can be used as a framework for **technical consultancy** by a wide range of international and national organizations that provide support to countries wishing to reform their mental health policy and/or services.

- They can be used as **advocacy tools** by consumer, family and advocacy organizations. The modules contain useful information for public education and for increasing awareness among politicians, opinion-makers, other health professionals and the general public about mental disorders and mental health services.

Format of the modules

Each module clearly outlines its aims and the target audience for which it is intended. The modules are presented in a step-by-step format so as to assist countries in using and implementing the guidance provided. The guidance is not intended to be prescriptive or to be interpreted in a rigid way: countries are encouraged to adapt the material in accordance with their own needs and circumstances. Practical examples are given throughout.

There is extensive cross-referencing between the modules. Readers of one module may need to consult another (as indicated in the text) should they wish further guidance.

All the modules should be read in the light of WHO's policy of providing most mental health care through general health services and community settings. Mental health is necessarily an intersectoral issue involving the education, employment, housing, social services and criminal justice sectors. It is important to engage in serious consultation with consumer and family organizations in the development of policy and the delivery of services.

Dr Michelle Funk   Dr Benedetto Saraceno

MENTAL HEALTH POLICY, PLANS AND PROGRAMMES

1. Introduction

An explicit mental health policy is an essential and powerful tool for the mental health section in any ministry of health. When properly formulated and implemented through plans and programmes, a policy can have a significant impact on the mental health of the population concerned. The outcomes described in the literature include improvements in the organization and quality of service delivery, accessibility, community care, the engagement of people with mental disorders and their carers, and in several indicators of mental health.

Despite wide recognition of the importance of national mental health policies, data collected by WHO reveal that 40.5% of countries have no mental health policy and that 30.3% have no programme (WHO, 2001b).

This module presents evidence-based guidance for the development and implementation of mental health policies, plans and programmes. The experiences of several countries are used as practical sources for drawing up mental health policies and implementing them through plans and programmes.

Mental health policy is commonly established within a complex body of health, welfare and general social policies. The mental health field is affected by many policies, standards and ideologies that are not necessarily directly related to mental health. In order to maximize the positive effects when mental health policy is being formulated it is necessary to consider the social and physical environment in which people live. It is also necessary to ensure intersectoral collaboration so that benefit is obtained from education programmes, health, welfare and employment policies, the maintenance of law and order, policies specifically addressing the young and the old, and housing, city planning and municipal services (WHO, 1987; WHO, 2001a).

The information provided in this module is considered relevant for various health systems, including those that are decentralized. It is generally accepted that national policy, plans and programmes are necessary in order to give mental health the appropriate priority in a country and to organize resources efficiently. Plans and programmes can be developed at the state, province, district, municipal and other local levels within countries in order to respond to specific local circumstances, while following national plans. If no overall national plan exists there is a risk of fragmentation or duplication of plans developed more locally.

The concepts and recommendations presented in this module are intended for countries and regions with a wide range of circumstances and resource levels. The module provides examples of how policy, plans and programmes can be developed for countries with low and medium resource levels.

2. Developing a policy: essential steps

It is important to have a time schedule in mind when approaching a mental health policy. It is probably realistic to allow one to two years for development and five to ten years for implementing and achieving changes (WHO, 1998a). Different elements of policy, plans and programmes may require different time scales.

Step 1. Gather information and data for policy development

Good policy is dependent on information about the mental health needs of the population and the mental health system and services offered. The needs of the population can be determined from, for example, prevalence and incidence studies, determining what communities identify as problems and an understanding of help seeking behaviour. Establishing priorities for mental health must also be done.

In addition, the current system for delivering mental health care must be well understood and documented. Knowing who delivers mental health, to whom and with what resources is an important starting point for developing a reasonable and feasible mental health policy.

Needs can be determined by the following methods:
   a) Formal research: Epidemiological studies in the general population
   and in special populations (e.g. schools and workplaces), simple epidemiological
   studies of people visiting health facilities, burden of disease studies involving
   the use of disability-adjusted life-years (DALYs), in-depth interviews
   and focus groups.
   b) Rapid appraisal: Secondary analysis of data from existing information systems,
   brief interviews with key informants and discussion groups involving people
   with mental disorders, families, carers and health staff.

Step 2. Gather evidence for effective strategies

Evidence can be obtained by visiting local services and reviewing the national
and international literature.
   a) Evidence from a country or region: The principal evidence comes
   from the evaluation of previous policy, plans and programmes. Pilot projects
   and local experiences are also excellent sources of information.
   b) Evidence from other countries or regions: Evidence can be gathered
   most usefully from countries or regions with similar cultural and socio-economic
   features.
   c) Evidence from the literature: Evaluations of national or regional mental
   health policies.

Step 3. Consultation and negotiation

The process of formulating and implementing a mental health policy is mainly political. To a lesser degree it is a matter of technical actions and resource-building. The role of the health ministry is to listen to the various stakeholders and to make proposals that blend their different views with the evidence derived from national and international experience. An active compromise of the majority of the key stakeholders may be required in order to develop and implement a mental health policy. It is very important to obtain political support.

Step 4. Exchange with other countries

Sharing experiences with other countries may help a country to learn about both the latest advances in more developed countries and about creative experiences and lower-cost interventions in less developed countries. International experts may also be helpful in this connection.

Step 5. **Set out the vision, values, principles and objectives**

When information has been gathered from a variety of sources through steps 1 to 4 the substance of the policy can now be set out by describing the vision, values, principles and objectives for mental health.

a) Vision: The vision usually sets high expectations for mental health, describing what is desirable for a country or region. However, it should be realistic, covering what is possible in accordance with the available resources and technology.

b) Values and principles: Different countries and regions have their own values associated with mental health and mental disorders. During the process of formulating mental health policy it is necessary to discuss which values and guiding principles should be adopted.

c) Mental health objectives: The three overall objectives of any health policy (WHO, 2000a) are applicable to mental health policy.

1. *Improving the health of the population*. The policy should clearly indicate the objectives for improving the mental health of the population. Ideally, mental health outcome indicators should be used, such as quality of life, mental functioning, disability, morbidity and mortality. If this is not possible, process indicators can also be used, such as access and service utilization.
2. *Responding to people's expectations*. In mental health this objective includes respect for persons and a client-focused orientation.
3. *Providing financial protection against the cost of ill-health*. Among the issues of relevance to mental health are: equity in resource distribution between geographical regions; availability of basic psychotropic drugs; parity of mental health services with those of general health; allocation of an appropriate percentage of the total health budget to mental health.

Step 6. **Determine areas for action**

The next step is to translate the objectives of the mental health policy into areas for action. In order to be effective a mental health policy should consider the simultaneous development of several such areas. The areas to include may vary in different countries and regions and in different historical periods. The following areas have been involved in most of the policies developed over the last 20 years.

- Financing
- Legislation and human rights
- Organization of services
- Human resources and training
- Promotion, prevention, treatment and rehabilitation
- Essential drug procurement and distribution
- Advocacy
- Quality improvement
- Information systems
- Research and evaluation of policies and services
- Intersectoral collaboration

Step 7. Identify the major roles and responsibilities of different sectors

The main sectors required to take on specific roles and responsibilities include:

- Governmental agencies (health, education, employment, social welfare, housing, justice);
- academic institutions;
- professional associations;
- general health and mental health workers;
- consumer and family groups;
- providers;
- nongovernmental organizations (NGOs);
- traditional health workers.

3. Developing a mental health plan

Step 1. Determine the strategies and timeframes

Strategies need to be determined for the different areas of action identified in Step 6 above and these strategies must then be co-ordinated to ensure that the plans are coherent and designed to meet the priority objectives. Strategies are generally formulated and prioritized through consultation with stakeholders and consideration of:

- the strengths and weaknesses of the established mental health system;
- the opportunities for and threats to the development of mental health policy and plans in the country or region concerned.

A time frame should be defined for each strategy. This means stating in what year each strategy will begin and for how long it will function. It is necessary for some strategies to keep functioning continuously and indefinitely. Others operate only for limited periods. It frequently happens that a strategy cannot be implemented in full as from the year when it begins because resources or capacities are inadequate.

Step 2. Set Indicators and targets

The strategies developed must be broken down into specific targets and indicators drawn up to later assess whether the plan has been effective or not. The targets must be clear and explicit and state precisely what must be achieved within given timeframes.

The targets must be measurable and indicators identified with respect to how the success of each target will be assessed.

Step 3. Determine the major activities

For each strategy, and in each area of action, detailed activities must be worked out with regard to how the strategy will be realized. A mental health plan needs to specify what activities will be taking place; who the people are who will take responsibility for each activity; how long each activity will take; when it will take place and which activities can be done simultaneously and which can only follow the completion of another. It is also necessary to specify what the expected outputs of each activity are as well as the potential obstacles and delays which could inhibit the realisation of the activity.

Step 4. **Determine the costs, available resources and budget accordingly**

A critical factor for the implementation of prioritized strategies is the availability of resources for mental health in the country or region. A mental health plan needs to:

- Calculate the costs of each strategy as well as the total costs of the plan for each year. The costs will include capital investments and recurrent costs such as human resources and consumables.
- Define who is going to finance these resources. At present, most countries have mixed structures for health financing, including different proportions of state funding (general taxation), social insurance, donors, private insurance and out-of-pocket payments. It is also important to consider that mental health requires expenditures from different government sectors in a country or region (education, labour, justice, housing, etc.), as well as from NGOs, consumer and family organizations, and private institutions.
- Adjust the time frames of the strategies and activities in accordance with what resources are available in different years.
- Replan the time frame and resources annually after monitoring and evaluation of the implementation of the plan.

4. Developing a mental health programme

In addition to the policy and strategic and detailed plans, it is important to have programmes for highly focussed objectives for the promotion of mental health, the prevention of mental disorders, and treatment and rehabilitation. A programme is frequently implemented in a smaller administrative division or for a shorter period than a strategic plan.

Programmes should focus on specific goals which are identified and require special attention for a particular reason at a particular time. For example, programmes may be designed and implemented in areas such as:

- Violence against women
- Fetal Alcohol Syndrome
- Refugees
- Secure mental health facilities
- World Health Day
- Treatment of epilepsy

Developing and implementing a programme cannot be done in a haphazard manner and should follow the steps outlined in plans. Programmes should hence track the following procedure:

> Determine strategies and time frames based on research and information collected
> Set indicators and targets
> Determine the major activities and how and by whom these will be implemented
> Determine the costs and available resources and orientate the programme accordingly
> Set up monitoring and evaluation processes

5. Implementation issues for policy, plans and programmes

A mental health policy can be implemented through the priority strategies identified by the plan and the priority interventions identified by the programme. Several actions are necessary in order to make possible the implementation of these strategies and interventions.

Step 1. Disseminate the policy

It is important that the ministry of health and the health districts disseminate the new policies widely to all the stakeholders.

Step 2. Generate political support and funding

After a policy has been written, active stakeholder participation and communication activities should be initiated. The goal of these activities is to ensure that enough political support and funding are provided for implementation. The country's leaders need to know that mental disorders represent a significant proportion of the burden of disease (DALYs) and that they generate important needs and demands. They should appreciate that there are effective strategies and that all sectors can contribute to the improvement of the people's mental health.

Step 3. Develop supportive organization

The implementation of mental health policy requires a competent group of professionals with expertise both in public health and mental health. This group should be responsible for managing the plan and programme(s). It should also be responsible for facilitating the active participation of consumers and families in all components of the mental health network and for establishing collaborative intersectoral actions.

> **At the level of the ministry of health:** A multidisciplinary team has proved very useful in several countries. The size of the team can vary from two part-time persons in small countries or regions to more than 10 full-time people in larger ones. The types of professionals to be considered include psychiatrists, public health physicians, psychologists, psychiatric nurses, social workers and occupational therapists.

> **At the level of the health district:** A mental health professional or, ideally, a multidisciplinary team similar to that at the ministry of health.

> **At the level of the community mental health teams:** It is highly recommended that each team have a coordinator who devotes a few hours a week to public health and management work.

> **At the level of the primary health care teams:** It is advisable that each primary care facility or team have a mental health coordinator.

Step 4. Set up pilot-projects in demonstration area(s)

The demonstration area can be a geographical region or a sector of a large city that is representative of the majority of the population of the country concerned. The knowledge that may be gained from a demonstration area is vital for the success of the policy in the whole country. It is also helpful as a training and orientation centre for district health staff.

Step 5. Empower mental health providers

Providers in a health system are teams or institutions that deliver health interventions to the population. Both general health providers and specific mental health providers deliver mental health interventions. Some interventions are provided by institutions outside the health sector.

The characteristics of providers may have a strong influence on the way in which mental health interventions are delivered. The ideal providers are small multidisciplinary teams comprising persons from different fields who combine their skills and use their collective wisdom in order to deal more effectively with the complexities of the population's mental health.

Six types of health providers can be differentiated, each requiring particular incentives:

- public mental health providers;
- private mental health providers;
- traditional health workers;
- mutual aid groups;
- nongovernmental, voluntary and charitable organizations;
- mental health consumers and families as providers.

Step 6. Reinforce intersectoral coordination

The tasks of the mental health professionals in the ministry of health are to:

> coordinate activities with professionals from other ministries in order to formulate, implement and evaluate mental health interventions conjointly;
> support mental health professionals in health districts to implement district intersectoral interventions;
> support mental health professionals in health districts to enhance coordination among local health teams and other sector teams.

Step 7. Promote interaction among stakeholders

In order to ensure the delivery of mental health interventions that respond to the needs of the population, multiple interactions have to take place among the different stakeholders. These interactions happen at different levels of the organization of a country or region.

5.7.1 Interaction between the ministry of health and other sectors

- Stakeholders with responsibility for funding: ministry of finance, social and private insurance, donor agencies and charitable organizations.

- Stakeholders with responsibility for provision: national organizations of providers, people with mental disorders and families, mutual aid groups, professional NGOs, health workers and traditional health workers.

- Stakeholders with responsibility for regulation: professional associations and advocacy groups.

5.7.2 Interaction between health districts and the ministry of health

One of the most important issues in this interaction is the degree of decentralization that the country or region requires in accordance with the general administrative structure, level of development of mental health services and social and cultural characteristics of the population.

> **Policy, plan and programme(s) at district or national/regional level:** Each country or region should evaluate the advantages and disadvantages of developing these at the central, district or local level, depending on the prevailing circumstances.

> **Allocation of funds from national or regional to district level:** Funds from the national or regional level can be allocated to the district level through various mechanisms.

> **Commissioning between health ministry and health districts:** The ministry agrees to transfer certain funds and technical support and the districts agree to deliver a certain volume of mental health interventions of a specified quality.

5.7.3 Interaction between health districts and providers

> **Management of mental health services:** Management can be implemented directly through the plan/programme(s) or indirectly through commissioning.

> **Purchasing of mental health services:** In this case the health district enters into a contract with a private provider in order to obtain a certain number of mental health interventions of a specified quality.

> **Regulation of mental health services:** Because districts can be providers it is to have multiple regulatory sources. This can be achieved by forming partnerships with consumer groups, family groups and mental health workers so as to build a culture of quality.

> **Coordination with other sectors delivering mental health interventions:** The professionals in charge of mental health in the health district should map the principal mental health services that are provided by institutions of other sectors. These may include mental health interventions conducted by other sectors, activities performed by health workers in order to complement other sectors, activities that health workers can implement in response to the needs of a population which have been detected by other sectors, and benefits that people with mental disorders can receive from other sectors.

5.7.4 Interaction between consumers and providers

> **Coordination of mental health services:** This can occur through regular meetings between primary health care teams and secondary mental health teams and between these health teams and representatives from other sectors.

> **Support for consumer and family groups:** In order to improve the accessibility and quality of mental health services and overcome the paternalistic attitudes of some providers, consumer and family organizations should be empowered.

> **Advocacy for mental health and mental disorders:** The stigma associated with mental health and mental disorders makes it necessary to develop an advocacy movement so as to produce a change in the local culture.

6. Recommendations and conclusions

Developing and implementing mental health policy, plans and programmes in a country or region is a complex process. Many factors have to be considered and the needs of multiple stakeholders have to be taken into account.

The specific circumstances of developing and implementing mental health policy, plans and programmes may vary enormously from one country to another. For each country, therefore, it is necessary to adapt the steps indicated in this module to the prevailing conditions.

Although there is variation between countries it is essential that countries develop policy, plans and programmes for mental health. A policy outlines a vision, values and principles; it identifies areas for action and indicates who will take responsibility for action; and it establishes priorities for strategies. A plan provides a detailed scheme for implementing strategic actions. A programme focuses on the design and implementation of specific objectives that need to be met to attain better mental health. Equipped with policies, plans and programmes, countries are in a good position to systematically improve the mental health of their populations.

The experience of several countries and regions shows that these steps or similar ones are feasible for the development and implementation of mental health policy, plans and programmes.

The whole process can produce positive mental health outcomes and the population of a country or region can receive the following benefits (WHO, 2001a):

- alleviation of symptoms associated with mental disorders;
- improvement of functioning in different areas (e.g. family, social, education, work);
- enhancement of productivity at work;
- improvement in the quality of life of persons with mental disorders and their families;
- prevention of psychological and social disability;
- reduction of mortality (e.g. suicide).

The process is complex and presents many obstacles. Nevertheless, improvements in the mental health, well-being, functioning and quality of life of people with mental disorders provides more than adequate motivation for the development and implementation of mental health policy, plans and programmes.

Aims	To present evidence-based guidance for the development and implementation of mental health policy, plans and programmes.
Target audience	Policy-makers and public health professionals of health ministries (or health offices) of countries and large administrative divisions of countries (regions, states, provinces).
How to use this module	The introduction lays the conceptual foundations for the module. Practical guidance is then provided for the formulation of mental health policy and the development of plans and programmes. A clear model for the implementation of policy, plans and programmes is set out, with case examples from specific countries. See Fig.1 for a visual outline of the process of developing and implementing mental health policy.

Countries or regions should adapt the guidance provided in this module to their specific circumstances. Examples are provided of how policies, plans and programmes can be developed and implemented in a variety of resource scenarios, particularly in countries with low and medium levels of mental health resource development.

Cross-references are frequently made to other modules in the Mental Health Policy and Service guidance package.

What is mental health policy?

Mental health policy is an organized set of values, principles and objectives for improving mental health and reducing the burden of mental disorders in a population. It defines a vision for the future and helps to establish a model for action. Policy also states the level of priority that a government assigns to mental health in relation to other health and social policies. Policy is generally formulated to cover a long period, e.g. 5 to 10 years.

Often the terms plans and programmes are used interchangeably. In this module they are considered complementary to policies and provide the means for implementing actions.

- **Mental health plan:** A detailed pre-formulated scheme for implementing strategic actions that favour the promotion of mental health, the prevention of mental disorders, and treatment and rehabilitation. Such a plan allows the implementation of the vision, values, principles, and objectives defined in the policy. A plan usually includes strategies, time frames, resources required, targets to be achieved, indicators and activities.

A plan can correspond to the same administrative division and period of time as the mental health policy. However, this does not always have to be so: a plan can be developed for a smaller administrative division or a shorter period than the policy.

- **Mental health programme:** An intervention or series of interventions with a highly focussed objective for the promotion of mental health, the prevention of mental disorders, and treatment and rehabilitation. A programme usually focuses on a specific mental health priority and, like mental health plans, programmes must be adequately designed, budgeted for, monitored and evaluated. In contrast to the policy and plan, the programme is frequently implemented in a smaller administrative division or for a shorter period.

The main differences between a mental health policy, a plan and a programme are summarized in Box 1. These concepts do not rigidly exclude each other: the borders between them are not clear-cut. In most countries there is frequently some overlapping between mental health policy, plans and programmes.

Mental health policy is an organized set of value principles and objective. improving mental healt. reducing the burden of . disorders in a populatio.

A mental health plan is a detailed pre-formulate. scheme for implementir strategic actions.

A mental health progran is a focused interventior achieving a specific, ofte short term goal.

Box 1. Some differences between mental health policy, plans and programmes

	Policy	Plans	Programmes
Focus	- Vision - Values - Principles - Broad objectives	- Strategies - Time frames - Financing - Human resources - Targets - Activities	- Specific interventions - Resources (physical and human) - Budget
Priority-setting	As between mental health and other health problems and between different mental health issues	Areas for action and types of strategies	Specific focus on identified short-term priorities
Scope of content	General	General or specific (according to strategies)	Specific
Duration	Long (5 to 10 years)	Medium (3 to 8 years)	Short (1 to 5 years)
Geographical area	Country or large division of country	Country to small division of country	Country to small local areas

Why is mental health policy important?

An explicit mental health policy is an essential and powerful tool for the mental health section in a ministry of health. WHO has recognized this fact for more than 30 years (WHO, 1984, 1987, 1996). In the field of mental health, **written policies are very important** for the following reasons:

> Policies provide a general blueprint, describe the broad objectives to be achieved and lay a foundation for future action.
> They give mental health a priority that is consistent with the disease burden that it represents and with the effectiveness of interventions in this field.
> They improve procedures for developing and prioritizing mental health services and activities.
> They identify the principal stakeholders in the mental health field and designate clear roles and responsibilities.
> They facilitate agreements for action among the different stakeholders.

Much has been learnt from the developments of mental health policy, plans and programmes in recent years. Equipped with a national mental health policy, plans and programmes, health ministries have had a significant impact on the mental health of populations in some countries. Some of the outcomes have been: improved organization and quality of service delivery; accessibility; community care; the engagement of both people with mental disorders and carers; and improvements in several indicators of mental health (Kemp, 1994; Cohen & Natella, 1995; De Jong, 1996; Commonwealth Department of Health and Family Services, Australia, 1997; Montejo & Espino, 1998; Thornicroft & Tansella, 1999; Barrientos, 2000). The absence of mental health policy and of a mental health section in a health ministry can have negative consequences (Pearson, 1992; Phillips, 2000).

Despite wide recognition of the importance of national mental health policy, 40.5% of countries have no mental health policy and 30.3% have no programme (WHO, 2001b). In addition, there has been enormous variation in the form and content of mental health policies and plans in different countries (Kemp, 1994).

How are policies normally formulated?

Mental health policy is commonly established within a complex body of health, welfare and general social policies. The mental health field is affected by many policies, standards and ideologies that are not necessarily directly related to mental health. In order to maximize the positive effects when formulating mental health policy it is necessary to consider the social and physical environment in which people live. It is also necessary to ensure intersectoral collaboration in order to benefit from: education programmes; health and welfare policies; employment policies; housing, city planning and municipal services; the maintenance of law and order; and policies specifically addressing the young or the old (WHO, 1987; WHO, 2001a).

There are many options for countries formulating a mental health policy, depending on cultural factors, political and social organization, and the importance given to mental health by governments. Some of the variables to consider are the institution responsible for the policy, the scope of the policy and the structure of the policy.

Institution responsible for mental health policy

Every government should have a mental health policy that is endorsed at the highest level. It is desirable that the policy be the responsibility of the **national government** for the following reasons:

> Mental health is closely related to human development and the quality of life.
> Mental disorders are highly prevalent and produce a significant burden of disease worldwide.
> The implementation of mental health interventions requires the participation of different sectors of the state.

In most countries the **ministry of health** is in charge of mental health policy. This has the advantage that the policy is implemented exclusively through one sector, thus favouring consistency and coherence. However, there are disadvantages in that the health sector cannot provide all the services needed by people with mental disorders and cannot address all requirements for the promotion of mental health and the prevention of mental disorders. These disadvantages can be partially overcome by creating a **national commission or council**, which, usually, is convened by the ministry of health and represents several stakeholders (welfare, religious, education, housing, labour, criminal justice, police and other social services).

In some countries the ministry of health has not endorsed a mental health policy, and the document is formulated and approved by the **mental health section or division**. In this case the policy has much less influence on the services delivered to the population, although it is still useful for prioritizing and organizing the executive functions expected from mental health teams at the different levels of the health system.

Scope of policy

Only a few countries have a **general** or **social policy** with some components of mental health. Where such a policy exists it usually focuses on mental health promotion. Whatever the content, the larger the scope of the policy the better it will be in terms of integrating mental health activities and services with other social services.

Most countries have either a **health policy** with a component of mental health or a specific **mental health policy**. The former is preferable because it favours the incorporation of promotion and prevention into the general approaches to health and decreases the risks of discrimination and stigmatization of people with mental disorders.

The scope of the mental health policy in many countries is restricted exclusively to **psychiatric services**. This has some advantages, e.g. a high degree of specificity and comparative ease of implementation and evaluation. However, this narrow focus does not allow for a more comprehensive response to the population's needs, e.g. aspects of mental health promotion and the prevention of disorders. The broader focus on **mental health services** usually covers both primary care and specialized care, with a mixture of promotion, prevention and rehabilitation, while psychiatric services can be limited mainly to the treatment of persons with mental disorders.

Structure of policy

There is great variability in the structure of mental health policies, plans and programmes. Some countries have only a **policy**, while others have formulated policy issues as part of a **mental health law** or a **reform** (either a general health reform or a reform of psychiatric services). If a mental health plan is not formulated at the same time in any of these cases, some elements of a plan are included in the policy. Other countries have produced a **mental health strategy**, a **mental health plan** or a **mental health programme** in which some elements of policy are incorporated.

No general recommendation can be made to guide the selection of any of these alternatives in a particular country or administrative division. The ultimate decision is the responsibility of government in accordance with considerations of history, culture, policies, the legal system, social structure, the type of health system and the meaning given to policy, plan and programme.

Regardless of the name and format of the policy, the important issue for government is to have a policy that is approved at the highest level and includes the core components described in this module.

What is the scope of this module?

The adequate advancement of mental health policy, plans and programmes in a country or region requires the following key steps:

Step 1: The development of mental health policy, plans and programmes.
Step 2: The implementation of the policy through the plans and programmes.
Step 3: The monitoring of implementation.
Step 4: Evaluation.
Step 5: The reformulation of the policy, plans and/or programmes.

This module deals mainly with the first two steps: developing and implementing policy, plans and programmes. Other modules deal with various aspects of steps 3, 4 and 5. *Planning and Budgeting for Service Delivery* addresses the development, monitoring and implementation of plans and budgets for services at the local or district level. *Quality Improvement* addresses the monitoring and evaluation of the quality of care. Modules to be developed by WHO will cover the national monitoring of policy, plans and programmes (*Information Systems*) and research and evaluation on policy, plans and programmes (*Research and Evaluation*) and other matters.

The information provided in this module is considered relevant for different health systems, including those that are decentralized. It is generally accepted that national policy, plans and programmes are necessary in order to give mental health a high priority in a country and to organize resources efficiently. States, provinces, districts, and municipal and other local levels can develop their own plans and programmes in order to respond to specific local circumstances, in accordance with national policy objectives, strategies and priorities. In the absence of an overall national plan there is a risk of fragmentation and/or duplication of plans developed at more local levels.

The concepts and recommendations presented in this module are intended for countries and regions with differing resources. As with the recommendations for action for three scenarios in Chapter 5 of the *World Health Report 2001* (WHO, 2001a), the present module gives guidance and examples for countries with low, medium and high levels of resources. Policies, plans and programmes can help to improve the mental health of populations across the entire resource spectrum.

Key points: Importance of mental health policy, plans and programmes

- A policy is an organized set of values, principles and objectives for improving mental health and reducing the burden of mental disorders in a population.

- A plan defines priority strategies, time frames, resources, targets and activities for implementing the policy.

- A programme focuses on specific mental health issues which require concentrated and usually shorter term interventions.

- Policy, plans and programmes can improve the quality of services, accessibility, community care, the participation of consumers and families, and the mental health level of populations.

2. Developing a mental health policy: essential steps

The experiences of various countries make it possible to identify several essential steps for the development of a successful mental health policy. Fig. 1 presents a framework of steps for developing a mental health policy, obtaining official approval and implementing the policy through plans and programmes. The framework is a visual summary of the contents of this module. The steps are described in more detail below.

It is important to have a **time schedule** in mind when approaching a mental health policy. One to two years for development and five to ten years for implementing and achieving changes are probably realistic periods (WHO, 1998a). A shorter time scale is likely to be impossible, while a time horizon that is too long may not satisfy many of the stakeholders and the general population. Different elements of policy, plans and programmes may require different time scales.

The persons in charge of mental health in the health ministry and health districts have to be competent, motivated and persistent in order to overcome the multiple obstacles that inevitably arise in this process (see Chapter 7 for examples of how to face obstacles).

A mental health policy takes approximately one to two years to develop and five to ten years to implement.

The persons in charge of mental health in the ministry and health districts have to be competent, motivated and persistent.

of the population, especially poor people, with little or no access to a mental health practitioner. Therefore it is important to map out the professionals available in both the private and public sector.

Another very important issue to "map" is the geographical distribution of human resources. It is common throughout the world for skilled professionals (including mental health practitioners) to be located mainly in urban areas. So while a country may seem to have adequate professionals relative to the population, this may hide the fact that in some areas accessibility and availability is extremely poor or even non-existent.

ii) Financial resources

In many countries there may be inadequate financial resources to meet the goals of the policy. Plans and programmes are also sometimes drawn up without careful consideration of what will be possible within the finances available. Obtaining additional resources for mental health is an important objective to improve services (see the module *Mental Health Financing*). Nonetheless in many countries mental health planners do not know how much is currently being spent on mental health, and the nature of the services which are being paid for. This can lead to futile preparation. Having reasonably accurate financial information is critically important for planning services.

In many countries the budget for mental health is distributed into various budget line items rather than the full mental health allocation being a separate "verticalized" allocation. For example mental health within primary care may be part of a district health service budget while psychiatric wards in general hospitals may be funded as part of a generalized hospital services budget. While we are not arguing here that all mental health services should be concentrated within a single mental health budget, a consequence of a spread budget is that it is difficult to rationally plan for mental health services and to prioritize based on need - and even on accepted policy. It is suggested that planners should know how much and where resources are spent, no matter which budget lines they are allocated from.

iii) Structure of service

When a new policy is developed it sometimes merely formalizes an existing way of providing services. More often though, a policy is developed in order to change the status quo. For change, planners need information on where and how services are being provided at a "base-line" or starting point.

A good understanding of the structure of services, combined with the information on human and financial resources and distribution described above, provides the necessary starting point for the detailed planning of services. For example, if most mental health services are provided within psychiatric institutions and the policy states that firstly services should be community oriented and secondly that prevention and promotion should be emphasized, planners can easily strategize on what services need to be closed down, what should be developed and so forth. Together with the baseline information on human and financial resources, planning hence becomes firmly reality-based.

iv) Views and attitudes of health workers

The best health policies and plans can fail if those who have to implement them are resistant to change it and/or to the particular change recommended.

As part of the assessment of "baseline" information necessary for making mental health plans, it may be important to understand the perspectives of health workers towards possible changes. This will provide guidance to planners on the difficulties that may be experienced in getting policy accepted and implemented.

It is necessary to have good data and understanding of the current situation with regard to the mental health system and provision of care.

Some of the "baseline" information mentioned in this section may be readily available and will require collation. On the other hand certain data will have to be acquired through conducting research. In the latter case it is important not to delay planning unnecessarily for detailed results to become available and rapid data collection methods may be appropriate.

Collection of data

The methods for gathering the above information can vary greatly depending on the resources and time available. Ways of collecting relevant information include formal research and rapid appraisal. While there is no categorical difference between formal research and rapid appraisal, the latter usually involves active participation of the services and the results become available to decision makers within days or weeks after the end of the survey. Formal research is usually more concerned with scientific rigour, for example sample size and use of standardized instruments, and is generally larger in scope and takes place over a longer period of time. Some examples are listed below.

a) Formal research

Epidemiological studies on the incidence and prevalence of mental disorders and the disabilities associated with them can be conducted either in the general population or in special populations (e.g. in schools, health facilities and workplaces). A WHO multisite study in primary care facilities is a good example of this (Üstün, 1995). Such studies can provide useful information but are generally expensive and require technology that is not always available in developing countries. In some cases, information obtained in one country can be extrapolated to others with similar cultural and social characteristics. (See the module *Planning and Budgeting to Deliver Services for Mental Health* for more details of this method.)

- Burden of disease studies (involving the use of DALYs) give very useful information permitting comparisons of mental disorders and physical illnesses by measures of early mortality and disability. They also allow for comparisons between different mental disorders.

- Qualitative studies based on in-depth interviews and focus groups can be a useful guide to the expectations of consumers regarding mental health services and to the degree of satisfaction with the care received (Arjonilla, Parada & Pelcastre, 2000).

- A study on the areas where finances are spent on mental health linked to equity and distribution may be extremely helpful to policy.

- Individual interviews and focus group discussions with health workers would enhance understanding of potential areas of resistance to policy changes and provide important information on the functioning and problems within the mental health service.

b) Rapid appraisal

Examples of information and methods to collect useful information for formulating policy and plans are listed below.

- Secondary analysis can be made of data available from the routine information system in the country concerned. Most countries have some information about mortality, admissions to hospitals, numbers of outpatient attendances and activities carried out in health facilities.

The information from brief interviews and discussion groups plus routine data from the health information system can be enough to formulate a mental health policy if the data are valid and reliable.

- Brief interviews with key informants and discussion groups involving people with mental disorders, families, carers and health staff provide useful information at low cost. The information obtained in this way, along with the data available from the health information system, can be enough to formulate a mental health policy if the data are valid and reliable.

- A "mapping" of all available resources within geographical areas and between the public and the private sectors may be carried out.

Step 2. Gather evidence for effective strategies

Once an assessment of the population's needs for mental health has been formulated it is necessary to gather evidence about effective strategies and interventions. Such evidence can be obtained by visiting local services within the country concerned, visiting other countries, and reviewing the national and international literature.

a) Evidence from within the country or region

Considering that some 60% of countries have a mental health policy and that some 70% have a programme (WHO, 2001b), the principal evidence comes from the evaluation of experiences gained in these countries. In countries or regions where a policy, plan or programme has been developed or implemented, the first step is to evaluate these processes.

The principal evidence c from the evaluation of th country's previous polic plans and programmes.

Pilot projects on mental health, especially those that have been evaluated, are an excellent source of information on which to base policy formulation. Successful and unsuccessful experiences can provide invaluable data. Examples of matters that could be dealt with in pilot projects include: the role of primary care in the prevention and early treatment of mental disorders, mental health promotion through sectors other than health, and community care for persons with severe mental disorders.

Besides pilot projects, there are several interesting experiences in mental health which can be described by general health and mental health teams, people with mental disorders, their families, NGOs and other sectors. Although most of these activities, particularly in developing countries, have not been formally designed or evaluated, they are certainly helping to improve the mental health of many people. The professionals in charge of mental health in the ministry of health should visit the facilities and programmes in the country or region concerned in order to learn about the best practices on which policy can be based.

There are several interes local experiences in me health on which to base policy.

b) Evidence from other countries or regions

Other countries or regions, especially those with similar cultural and socio-economic features, can also provide examples of best practices in mental health. In particular, countries or regions that have formulated and/or implemented mental health policy and plans can be sources of useful information.

c) Evidence from the literature

By reviewing the literature it is possible to learn lessons from evaluations of national or regional mental health policies. See the "Further reading" section of this module for examples such evaluations (Commonwealth Department of Health and Family Services, Australia, 1997; Cohen & Natella, 1995; De Jong, 1996; Goering, Cochrane, Lesage et al., 1997; Montejo & Espino, 1998; Planning Commission, Pakistan, 1998).

Other countries or regions and the literatur can provide lessons abc national or regional mer health policies.

Step 3. **Consultation and negotiation**

The process of developing mental health policy is largely political. To a lesser degree it involves technical actions and resource-building. Many individuals, organizations and communities participate, each with particular values, interests, power bases, strengths and weaknesses. Many interactions, struggles and negotiations can be expected to occur.

From the point of view of the mental health professionals in a health ministry it is not enough to define vision, objectives and areas for action, or to formulate a plan with priorities and resources. Nor is it sufficient that the government provides funding, since this can be wasted or can produce powerlessness and dependency if insufficient attention is paid to developing local capacities, participation processes and alliances with different stakeholders.

In order for a mental health policy to be successful the health ministry should concern itself with consultation and negotiation at each stage. Policy has the potential to involve people and give them ownership of the mental health issues that affect them. The development of any policy can begin at the top or from the grass roots. If it originates at the top, without support from stakeholders, it will be difficult to implement later on. The community needs opportunities to deliberate about the values and principles associated with mental health and to consider various strategies that may prove reasonable for meeting them (Driscoll, 1998).

One of the most difficult processes is that of achieving a **common vision** among stakeholders from diverse backgrounds. Part of the problem is that different stakeholders interpret the mental health needs of populations in different ways. Moreover, many definitions of mental health are given in the literature. Some authors argue that mental health is a positive state of mind, emotions and behaviours, which should be promoted and protected by actions from different sectors. For other authors, the issue of mental health requires a focus on mental disorders, and associated issues of treatment and rehabilitation in the health sector.

The role of the health ministry in this process is to listen to the various stakeholders and to make proposals that blend their different views with the evidence derived from national and international experience. An **active compromise among the majority of the key stakeholders** may be necessary in order to develop and implement the mental health policy.

The mental health professionals in the ministry of health should have an active role in inviting stakeholders to be involved in the formulation and implementation of the new policy. (See Box 2 for examples of stakeholders.) Everyone can contribute to this process from her or his particular position in society.

The process of developing mental health policy is largely political.

The community needs the opportunity to deliberate about the values and principles related to mental health.

One of the most difficult processes is that of achieving a common vision among stakeholders from diverse backgrounds.

The ministry of health should invite stakeholders to involve themselves in the formulation and implementation of the new policy.

Box 2. Examples of stakeholders who may be invited for consultation about mental health policy, plans and programmes*

- **Consumer and family groups:** representatives or associations of persons with mental disorders and their families, mutual help groups, advocacy organizations representing the interests of people with mental disorders.

- **General health and mental health workers:** representatives from different types of general health and mental health facilities, as well as trade unions and other organizations that represent their interests.

- **Providers:** managers and administrators of public and private services and institutions concerned with general health and mental health.

- **Government agencies:** including heads of government and ministries of internal affairs, finance, trade and industry, justice, police, health, education, employment (labour), environment, housing, and social welfare, and local governments, municipalities and parliaments.

- **Academic institutions:** especially those that train psychiatrists, psychologists, nurses, social workers, other health professionals and technicians.

- **Professional associations:** such as those of psychiatrists, psychologists, general practitioners, nurses, occupational therapists and social workers.

- Profit and not-for-profit professional **nongovernmental organizations (NGOs):** including those involved in a variety of work related to mental health and those specifically providing care, treatment and rehabilitation services to persons with mental disorders.

- **Traditional health workers:** healers associated with traditional, religious and alternative systems of health.

- **Religious organizations**

- Other special interest groups such as **minority organizations**, including groups representing indigenous ethnic minorities.

- Other people and groups, e.g. national and local leaders, politicians, political parties, trade unions and the business community.

* the examples are not specific recommendations for action.

It is very important that the mental health professionals in the ministry of health obtain **political support** for the development of mental health policy. This means making the relevant authorities aware of the magnitude of the burden of mental disorders in their country, the strength of the needs and demands of the population, and the cost-effectiveness of several mental health interventions.

It is worth considering the development of a communication plan in order to support the idea of writing a national mental health policy. There is great value, for example, in placing negative stories in the media about the inadequacies of current policy and services, as well as positive stories about what would be attainable if a new mental health policy were developed. This can often be done with the support of people with mental disorders, their families and nongovernmental organizations.

Another strategy for obtaining political support involves identifying issues considered to be priorities by political leaders and offering the contribution of mental health interventions. Among such issues are those of interpersonal violence, drug trafficking, dissatisfaction with health services, and the rights of people with disabilities. If one of these subjects is chosen for a national policy a mental health component can be incorporated (Freeman, 2000).

Policy is a struggle for influence. It should be seen in the context of differing ideologies and should be related to the structure and organization of society as a whole. The development of a mental health policy and plan requires that a broad array of community elements be in active play. Driscoll (1998) suggested including a champion of the cause, a working group that does the background work and uses a collaborative approach, politicians, public service staff, opinion leaders, the media, the community at large, external elements, and a process of review and evaluation.

Step 4. Exchange with other countries

Because of the rapid development of mental health policies throughout the world it is very useful for health ministries in different countries to exchange information. The sharing of experiences can lead to countries learning about the latest advances from more developed countries and about creative experiences and lower-cost interventions from less-developed countries.

International experts may be helpful in the first stages of the formulation of mental health policies. Their knowledge of several countries enables them to recommend a broad range of solutions to the mental health needs of populations and to validate local pilot experiences. The possibility of adopting new strategies and new interventions may emerge when such experts are consulted. At the stage of policy implementation, international experts can make visits and provide external feedback in order to help the ministry of health to evaluate change.

Professionals in charge of mental health in the ministry of health need to keep in touch with their counterparts in other countries, particularly those with similar cultural and social backgrounds. They should also maintain close relationships with international agencies, especially WHO, which can supply them with technical support.

The mental health professionals in the ministry of health should obtain political support for the development of policy.

People with mental disorders, families and NGOs can provide support for the idea of a new policy.

Policy is a struggle for influence.

It is useful for ministries of health to exchange information about policy with other countries.

Step 5. **Set out the vision, values, principles and objectives of the policy**

It is possible to begin determining the main content of mental health policy once the population's needs have been identified, evidence for effective policies has been gathered, and the consultation process is under way.

The *World Health Report 2000* (WHO, 2000a) identified three objectives for health policies. These can be used as a framework for determining the vision, values, principles and objectives of mental health policy.

- **Improving the health of the population:** This is the primary or defining objective of a health system. Other sectors in a country may contribute towards achieving better health for a population but this is not their primary goal.

- **Responding to people's expectations:** This social objective, common to many sectors, concerns the way in which individuals or groups in society wish to be treated by particular facilities or services.

- **Providing financial protection against the cost of ill-health:** This objective is shared by all societal systems. It has to do with fair financing, whether the health system is paid for socially or financed by individual purchases. Prepayment, either through general taxation or social or private insurance, is preferable to out-of-pocket payment.

2.5.1 Determining the vision for mental health policies

The vision of the mental health policy represents a general image of the future of mental health care in a given population. This usually includes the type of services that are required and the way in which they will be financed. The vision usually sets high expectations as to what is desirable for a country or region in the realm of mental health. At the same time it should be realistic, taking account of what is possible with reference to the available resources and technology. The main elements of a mental health policy should be blended into a description of the final stage which will be reached after years of successful implementation. The vision also needs to motivate the different stakeholders of the country or region in question, touching some of their emotional sensibilities and impelling them to make their best efforts in order to achieve a higher level of mental health for the people.

The vision represents a general image of the future of mental health, the type of services and their financing.

The vision needs to motivate the different stakeholders of the country or region.

In South Africa, for example, the vision for mental health is that a comprehensive and community-based mental health service should be planned and coordinated at the national, provincial, district and community levels, and that it should be integrated with other health services (Department of Health of South Africa, 1997). In this example the vision for the transformation of the mental health system includes:

> a community-based service;
> a comprehensive, integrated service;
> a performance-driven service;
> an affordable service;
> adequate resources and decision-making power for those who plan and manage mental health services;
> the need to monitor the quality of care in hospitals and the community, associated with increased concern for the rights and needs of patients.

2.5.2 Values and principles in mental health policies

Values and principles are the base on which governments set objectives and goals and develop strategies and courses of action. Although not always explicitly formulated in policy documents, they nevertheless underlie all policy statements.

Countries, regions, and cultural and social groups within countries have their own values associated with mental health and mental disorders. During the process of formulating mental health policy it is necessary to discuss which values and guiding principles should be adopted. This has to be done both at the national level and in the administrative divisions of the country concerned. The process should strike a balance between common values and principles on the one hand and the realities imposed by stakeholders' and countries' cultural, social and economic circumstances on the other. The professionals in the ministry of health should refer consistently to these values and principles in order to foster greater coherence, integrity, comprehensiveness and continuity in the implementation of mental health policy.

As a consequence of the development of the mental health advocacy movement in many countries, people of different nationalities share some values and principles of mental health policies (See the module *Advocacy for Mental Health*).

Box 3 lists some examples of values and principles that are included in the mental health policies of various countries, states and provinces.

Values and principles are the base on which governments set objectives.

The ministry of health should refer consistently to values and principles in order to foster greater coherence, integrity, comprehensiveness and continuity of policy.

Box 3. Examples of values and principles in mental health policies*
(WHO, 1987; WHO, 1996; Ministry of Supply and Services, Canada, 1988;
Mental Health Division, Alberta Health, Canada, 1993; Planning Commission,
Pakistan, 1998; Department of Health, UK, 1999; Thornicroft & Tansella, 1999;
Freeman, 1999; Ministry of Health, Chile 2000).

1. Improving the health of the population

Values	Principles
PSYCHOLOGICAL WELL-BEING	- Mental health promotion should be integrated into social and educational services. - There should be intersectoral collaboration and linkage with community development.
MENTAL HEALTH INDIVISIBLE FROM GENERAL HEALTH	- Mental health should be integrated into the general health system. - Persons with mental disorders should be admitted to general hospitals.
COMMUNITY CARE	- People with mental disorders should be cared for in facilities with the least restrictive form of care. - The provision of community care alternatives should be tried before inpatient care is undertaken.

2. Responding to people's expectations

Values	Principles
COMMUNITY PARTICIPATION	- People with mental disorders should be involved in the planning, delivery and evaluation of services. - Mutual aid and advocacy groups should be encouraged.
CULTURAL RELATIVISM	- Different cultures should contribute their visions. - Traditional healers and informal sectors should play a significant role.
PROTECTION OF VULNERABLE PEOPLE	- The human rights of persons with mental disorders should be protected. - Women, children, elderly people and the very poor should be targets of specific mental health strategies.

3. Providing financial protection

Values	Principles
ACCESSIBILITY AND EQUITY	- Services should be accessible to all people, regardless of their geographical location, economic status, race or social condition. - Mental health services should have parity with general health services.

* the examples are not specific recommendations for action.

The three overall objectives of any health policy (WHO, 2000a) can be equally applied to the formulation of objectives for mental health policy.

- **Improving the health of the population:** The policy should clearly set out its objectives for improving the mental health of the population. Ideally, mental health outcome indicators should be used, such as quality of life, mental functioning, disability, morbidity and mortality. In developing countries, however, information systems are generally poorly developed and ministries of health may have to use some process indicators, e.g. access and service utilization.

- **Responding to people's expectations:** In mental health this objective can relate to both, respect for persons (human rights, dignity, confidentiality, and autonomy with respect to choice) and client-focused orientation (patient satisfaction, prompt attention, quality of amenities, access to social support networks and choice of provider).

- **Providing financial protection against the cost of ill-health:** Among the issues of relevance to mental health are equity in the distribution of resources between geographical regions, availability of basic psychotropic medication, parity of mental health services with general health services, and the allocation of an appropriate percentage of the health budget to mental health.

Some examples of mental health objectives which are formulated in line with the three above factors are listed below.

- Discharge patients from institutional care to comprehensive community based programmes (deinstitutionalization)
- Provide evidence based and cost-effective treatment to all people who need mental health care
- Promote the human rights of people with mental disabilities
- Integrate mental health into general health care
- Promote good mental health through sectoral and intersectoral initiatives
- Prevent mental disorders through mental health promotion activities

Objectives: improving health, responding to expectations and providing financial protection.

Key points: Content of mental health policy

- **Vision:** sets what is desirable for the mental health of a country or region and what is possible in accordance with the available resources and technology.

- **Values and principles:** build the base on which governments set objectives and goals and develop strategies and courses of action.

- **Objectives:** improving the health of the population, responding to people's expectations and providing financial protection against the cost of ill-health.

Step 6. Determine areas for action

The next step is to translate the objectives of the mental health policy into areas for action. In order to be effective a mental health policy should consider the simultaneous development of several such areas. The areas that should be included may vary between countries or regions and between historical periods. However, some common areas can be identified in most of the policies developed over the last 20 years. They are listed in Box 4 and described in greater detail subsequently.

The policy should incorporate some actions in most of these areas, although the emphasis given to each one may differ from one country or region to another. The selection of areas and strategies should be based on the information obtained from all the previous steps of policy development.

A mental health policy
should consider the
simultaneous developme
of several areas for actio

Box 4. Principal areas for action in mental health policy

1. Financing

2. Legislation and human rights

3. Organization of services

4. Human resources and training

5. Promotion, prevention, treatment and rehabilitation

6. Essential drug procurement and distribution

7. Advocacy

8. Quality improvement

9. Information systems

10. Research and evaluation of policies and services

11. Intersectoral collaboration

2.6.1 Financing

As described in the *Financing* module, adequate and sustained financing is one of the most critical factors in the implementation of a mental health policy. Financing is the mechanism whereby resources are allocated for infrastructure, technology, the delivery of services and the development of a trained workforce. As such it is a powerful tool allowing the ministry of health to translate policy into reality and to develop and shape mental health services and their outcomes.

Every government should move progressively towards adequate funding for mental health, commensurate with the magnitude and burden of the mental disorders present in the society concerned. The amount of resources available for mental health is critical. Equally important is how they are allocated between regions, different segments of the population, and different services and programmes. Mental health professionals in the ministry of health should provide guidance and make decisions on the distribution of funding within the mental health system, defining which services are covered and which receive priority.

Adequate financing is on
of the most critical factor
in the implementation of
a mental health policy.

Every government shoulc
move progressively towa
adequate funding for
mental health.

The general characteristics of good financing for mental health are described in the *World Health Report 2001* (WHO, 2001a). They include protecting people from catastrophic financial risk caused by service costs and distributing the financial burden so that the healthy members of society subsidize those in need of services and so that the affluent subsidize the poor. Prepayment systems that include mental health services, e.g. general taxation and social insurance, are a clear way of achieving these objectives.

Mental health policy should include decisions about the allocation of resources. Following are some questions that have to be answered in this connection.

- *Type of service*. Which services are given funding priority (hospital vs. community care; primary care vs. specialized care, promotion/prevention vs. treatment/rehabilitation)? Are priorities given to service access at the cost of service quality?

- *Target population*. Are particular groups in the population given special priority (children vs. adults; persons with less severe disorders vs. persons with severe mental disorders; the general population vs. vulnerable groups such as abused women, the elderly, the extremely poor, persons with disabilities, victims of war, indigenous ethnic minorities, migrants)?

- *Geographical region*. Do particular geographical areas have special needs (urban vs. rural areas, areas where persons with mental disorders are underserved vs. areas where natural disasters have placed people at increased risk)?

See the *Financing* module for a more detailed discussion of these issues.

2.6.2 Legislation and human rights

The development of a mental health policy can promote or violate human rights, depending on the way in which it is formulated or implemented. Mental health legislation (as described in the *Legislation and Human Rights module*) should codify and consolidate the fundamental principles, values and objectives of mental health policy. Such legislation is essential in order to guarantee that the dignity of patients is preserved and that their fundamental human rights are protected (WHO, 2001a).

Some of the components to consider for legislation are indicated below. (See module entitled *Legislation and Human Rights* for details.)

- *The rights of persons with mental disorders in the health sector*: the least restrictive care that is possible, confidentiality, informed consent, voluntary and involuntary admission, voluntary and involuntary treatment, periodic review mechanism, competence.

- *The rights of persons with mental disorders in sectors outside health*: housing, employment, social security, criminal justice and civil legislation.

- *The promotion of mental health and the prevention of mental disorders*: parental bonding with neonates, mental health in primary care, child abuse and domestic violence, restriction of access to alcohol and drugs, indigenous ethnic minorities.

The field of mental health has a great need for human rights legislation. Various barriers make it difficult for persons with mental disorders to receive the care and treatment that they need. Once they obtain such care there is a high risk that their needs will not be met and that their rights will be abused. The risk is higher than the corresponding risk to which persons with a physical illness are subjected. In addition there are many barriers to the implementation of preventive interventions for mental disorders and to the promotion of mental health. Laws can help to overcome many of these barriers.

Legislation can help to enhance services through the definition of standards of mental health care, both in primary and specialist services. Evidence-based practice guidelines, developed by ministries of health and health districts in collaboration with the appropriate professional bodies, can complement legal provisions.

2.6.3 Organization of services

The organization of services is another critical area of mental health policy because services are the means whereby policy reaches people. Services are responsible for implementing programmes through the delivery of effective mental health interventions. Adequately organized services can greatly help towards achieving the objectives of policy. (See the module *Organization of Services for Mental Health*.)

According to the *World Health Report 2001* (WHO, 2001a) the three major strategies for facilitating the development of an effective network of mental health services are: shifting care away from large psychiatric hospitals; developing community mental health services; and integrating mental health care into general health services. (For further details see the module *Organization of Services for Mental Health*.)

> *Shifting care away from large psychiatric hospitals*: In many developing countries the principal resource for many years was a large psychiatric hospital. Fortunately, this situation has been changing over recent years. Efforts have been made in many places to transform the hospital resources into community mental health services (Alarcon & Aguilar-Gaxiola, 2000). For instance, ambulatory rehabilitation programmes, day care centres and sheltered homes have been created for persons with long-term severe mental disorder.

> *Developing community mental health services*: Several developed countries have demonstrated that deinstitutionalization is possible through the development of comprehensive community services. This has led to improvements in clinical outcomes, in the level of satisfaction with services and in the quality of life (Health Canada, 1998). These community services include:

- case management and assertive community treatment
  for persons with severe mental disorders;
- 24-hour crisis intervention services;
- day hospitals as alternatives to inpatient treatment;
- domiciliary treatment;
- supported housing;
- vocational rehabilitation and supported employment;
- opportunities for daytime activities;
- support services for consumer and mutual aid initiatives and organizations;
- support services for family initiatives and organizations.

> **Integrating mental health care into general health services**: Such integration has many advantages, such as reduced stigmatization of persons with mental disorders and a more efficient use of health resources. Integration can be achieved in both primary care centres and in general hospitals. Efforts should be made by professionals in charge of mental health in health districts to educate health staff about mental disorders. This helps to prevent stigmatization in general health facilities.

Experience gained in many countries shows that links between primary and secondary health care are necessary in order to develop accessible and effective mental health services. These links consist of shared time devoted to the discussion of cases, the assessment of patients with multiple problems, agreement on clinical guidelines, learning new psychological skills, improving referral and counter-referral mechanisms and defining administrative issues.

Legislation can help to enhance services by defining standards of mental health care.

Services are responsible for delivering effective mental health interventions.

Efforts have been made to transform mental hospital resources into community services.

Comprehensive community services improve clinical outcomes, satisfaction with services and the quality of life.

The integration of mental health services into general health services decreases stigmatization and allows a more efficient use of resources.

Links between primary and secondary care help to develop accessible and effective services.

2.6.4 Human resources and training

Human resources are the most important assets of the mental health system. The performance of the health care system depends ultimately on the knowledge, skills and motivation of the people responsible for delivering services (WHO, 2000a). Governments can consider different alternatives for developing human resources in their mental health policies, depending on the resources available for mental health and educational institutions. Cultural and social factors, as well as general health policies, must be taken into consideration when these strategies are being formulated.

In order to develop appropriate mental health policies it is necessary to determine the present number and type of human resources. It is also necessary to make a projection of the resources required for the near future (e.g. in 5 or 10 years). (See the module *Human Resources and Training*, to be developed by WHO.)

Policy should determine the present number and type of human resources and should make a projection for the future.

There is wide variation in the categories and numbers of people engaged in mental health workforces. The following types are the most likely to be involved with mental health (WHO, 2001a):

- general physicians;
- neurologists and psychiatrists;
- community and primary health care workers;
- allied mental health professionals, such as nurses, occupational therapists, psychologists and social workers);
- traditional health workers.

2.6.5 Promotion, prevention, treatment and rehabilitation

Comprehensive mental health policy should include a broad spectrum of actions ranging from promotion to rehabilitation. There is evidence of the effectiveness of a number of interventions in primary and secondary prevention (WHO, 1999; WHO, 2001a).

Comprehensive mental health policy should include a broad spectrum of actions ranging from promotion to rehabilitation.

A number of entry points for promotion can be defined in a mental health policy. The most appropriate entry point depends on information derived from needs' assessment and the social, cultural, gender, age-related and developmental contexts of specific countries. Actions in this area include those that target:

- factors determining or maintaining mental ill-health, for example, poverty and stigma;
- population groups, for example whole populations or population subgroups defined by age, gender, specific risk or vulnerability;
- the setting where the interventions take place, i.e. workplaces, schools, health services and families;
- particular health problems, behaviours or specific mental disorders.

Mental health promotion, the prevention of mental disorders, and treatment and rehabilitation are complementary strategies in mental health policy. They are all essential for achieving positive outcomes. However, mental health promotion is, even more than care and the prevention of mental disorders, an intersectoral responsibility, where education, work, justice, housing and other social areas should play a major role.

Mental health promotion is, even more than prevention and care, an intersectoral responsibility.

Ministries of health have much more experience in formulating mental health policies on prevention, treatment and rehabilitation than on promotion. The *World Health Report 2001* (WHO, 2001a) presents a good summary of the type of evidence on prevention, treatment and rehabilitation available for depression, alcohol dependence, drug dependence, schizophrenia, epilepsy, dementia, intellectual disability, hyperkinetic disorders and suicide (Box 19, Annex 1).

2.6.6 Essential drug procurement and distribution

Given the significant progress that has been achieved in the management of severe and disabling mental disorders through the utilization of psychotropic drugs, it is desirable to incorporate their purchase and distribution into a mental health policy. Their use has not only contributed to a significant reduction in hospitalization and to a much greater emphasis on community care but has also considerably reduced human suffering and improved the quality of life.

Psychotropic drugs hav' a considerable impact ir reducing human suffer and improving the quality of life.

Essential drugs are those considered indispensable and necessary for the mental health needs of the population. They should be restricted to those proven to be therapeutically effective, acceptably safe, and affordable in accordance with the level of resources of the country or region concerned (WHO, 1993a, 1993b). A module on *Improving Access and Use of Psychotropic Medicines* is to be developed by WHO.

Five essential steps that have been outlined for facilitating the rational use of psychotropic drugs in primary health care (WHO, 1993b) can be applied to specialized care:

- *Focus on a limited number of conditions*: This facilitates the training of health workers and the implementation of the programmes.

- *Make a limited range of drugs available*: This is helpful for bulk purchase or local man- ufacture, allowing a relatively cheap and constant supply and adequate quality control.

- *Simplify the division of tasks in connection with the use of drugs*: This helps to facilitate the delegation of some aspects of prescription and dispensing from physicians and pharmacists to other members of health teams.

- *Establish a continuous training programme*: This helps to improve adherence to and the effectiveness of drug treatment.

- *Set up a central policy body*: This contributes to the development of safeguards and regulations for improving the quality of treatments and limiting the abuse of drugs.

2.6.7 Advocacy

There is increasing evidence that consumer participation in advocacy and mutual help organizations can have positive outcomes (Health Canada, 1998). Among these outcomes are a decrease in the duration of inpatient treatment and in the number of visits to health services, as well as reinforcement of knowledge and skills. Other possible beneficial effects are increased self-esteem, an improved sense of well-being, improved coping skills, the reinforcement of social support networks, and improvements in family relationships.

There is evidence that consumer participation in advocacy may have several positive outcome

Consumers, families and advocacy groups can have a significant influence on the development of mental health policy. Examples of their roles are indicated below (Ministry of Health, Chile, 2000).

- They can make national authorities, community authorities and the media aware of the importance of mental disorders in the country concerned.
- They can identify and communicate public needs and expectations about mental health services.
- They can provide advocacy for patients' rights, including respectful treatment and service access.
- They can exercise social pressure in order to obtain more and better mental health services and social services.

- They can deliver mutual help and support as well as psycho-education.
- They can become leaders for cultural change in favour of eliminating discrimination and of social placements and work insertion.
- They can provide rehabilitation services for people with mental disabilities.

Policy should acknowledge that health ministries play an important role in advocacy. (See the module *Advocacy for Mental Health*.) They can implement advocacy actions directly, thereby influencing the mental health of the general population and the rights of persons with mental disorders. At the same time, ministries of health may achieve an impact on these populations indirectly, through supporting consumer, family and nongovernmental organizations dedicated to advocacy. Moreover, by working with the media it is possible for health ministries to carry out many advocacy activities.

Policy should acknowledge that ministries of health play an important role in advocacy.

2.6.8 Quality improvement

In order to be effective a mental health policy should place some emphasis on quality improvement. This is essential for the production of positive outcomes in mental health promotion, preventive activities, and the treatment and rehabilitation of persons with mental disorders. A quality orientation also results in the optimal use of limited resources and can reduce the overuse and misuse of services. Ongoing quality monitoring provides an in-built mechanism for continually improving the effectiveness and efficiency of policy, plans and programmes.

A quality orientation results in positive outcomes and optimal use of limited resources.

Governments should introduce specific tools for maintaining, monitoring and improving quality as part of their mental health policy. Some of these tools are indicated below. (Details are given in the module *Quality Improvement for Mental Health*.)

- Accreditation of providers and organizations.
- Standards for programmes, facilities and services.
- Clinical guidelines (development, dissemination, implementation).
- Measurement of performance (including consumer and family member perspective).
- Continuous quality improvement.
- Monitoring of outcomes.
- Consumer and family education.

WHO has contributed to this process with several documents, most notably *Quality assurance in mental health care: checklists and glossaries* (WHO, 1994). This type of document can help ministries of health and health districts to ensure that persons with mental disorders receive appropriate care in different facilities. (See also the module *Quality Improvement for Mental Health*.)

2.6.9 Information systems

The formulation of a policy should be based on up-to-date and reliable information concerning the community, mental health indicators, effective treatments, prevention and promotion strategies, and mental health resources. The policy should be reviewed periodically in order to allow for the modification or updating of programmes (WHO, 2001a).

A mental health information system should be developed in consultation with consumers and families so as to meet concerns about confidentiality and to develop sensible procedures for accessing information. Common standards in information technology allow local information systems to communicate across agency and geographical boundaries as people with mental disorders move around.

Professionals in charge of mental health in health ministries and health districts should develop a common basic information system in accordance with the level of resources and technical capacity of the country or district concerned. This makes data available for the monitoring and evaluation of policy. A module on *Information Systems* is to be developed by WHO.

Examples of mental health indicators are:

- The magnitude of risk factors for mental health, e.g. use of alcohol and drugs, number of victims of violence in the home, etc.;
- The rate of mental disorders, i.e. incidence and prevalence rates, diagnosis at discharge from hospital and/or when consulting at primary health care or specialist facilities;
- The consequences of mental disorders, i.e. disability and mortality rates;
- The numbers of human and physical resources, i.e. primary care workers trained in mental health, mental health professionals and staff, hospital beds, places in day hospitals, halfway houses and sheltered homes, medication;
- The quality of services, i.e. the extent to which facilities and programmes meet standards, prescription patterns, compliance rates, involvement in rehabilitation programmes;
- The efficiency of service utilization, i.e. the numbers of hospital admissions and re-admissions, the average duration of admissions, bed occupancy, outpatient attendance, consumers on case registers, filled day-service places;
- Costs, i.e. intervention costs (e.g. one day in hospital, one day in a sheltered home, one session with a health worker), facility operating costs, capital costs, transport costs, overheads;
- Outcomes, i.e. symptom relief, quality of life, level of functioning, consumer satisfaction, defaulter rate, relapse rates.

2.6.10 Research on and evaluation of policy and services

Investment in research and the wider dissemination of findings are important for extending knowledge about the magnitude and causes of mental disorders and about the possibilities for prevention, improved treatments and services. Although knowledge about these subjects has increased over the last decade there are still many unknown variables (WHO, 1998b; WHO 2001a).

The *World Health Report 2001* (WHO, 2001a) describes the principal areas for mental health research that can be considered within the development of a policy. They are as follows:

> Epidemiological data are essential for assessing the mental health of populations, identifying risk and protective factors, setting priorities and evaluating public health interventions. They are also important for advocacy.

> Research on treatment, prevention and promotion outcomes is needed for the development of more effective and cost-effective pharmacological, psychological and psychosocial interventions. More knowledge is required in order to understand what intervention works best and for whom.

> Research on policy and services is needed in order to guide mental health system reforms and deinstitutionalization, especially in developing countries. Other priority subjects for research in this area are the impact of different training strategies for mental health providers, treatment outcomes for traditional healing practices, and the effects of different policy decisions on access, equity and treatment outcomes.

> There is a need for more research on the costs of mental disorders and for economic evaluations of treatment, prevention and promotion programmes.

A basic information sys makes data available for the monitoring and evaluation of policy.

A set of mental health indicators is needed.

Research can extend knowledge about the magnitude and causes of mental disorders and about the possibilities for prevention, improve treatments and services

> There are great needs for mental health research in developing countries on which to base policies. There are also needs for international comparisons in order to improve understanding of the commonalties and differences in the management of mental disorders across different cultures.

Policy can define priorities for mental health research in response to the principal needs of a population. Some strategies that could be considered are:

- To identify a percentage of research funding for mental health within the general funds for health research;

- to encourage the training of mental health research professionals, including the provision of fellowships in developed countries;

- to support the development of national mental health research centres in universities and similar institutions;

- to establish collaborative research initiatives with more developed countries and international agencies.

2.6.11 Intersectoral collaboration

Several sectors outside health provide services that affect people's mental health. Policy should take account of these services and their impact on mental health. They include services provided by welfare, religious, education, housing, employment, criminal justice, police and other social services. Intersectoral collaboration also includes services within workplaces, such as those for human resource management, training and occupational health and safety, all of which influence mental health.

Several sectors outside health provide services that affect people's mental health levels.

Most mental health policies should incorporate a distribution of rights and responsibilities between different ministries. Some important examples of intersectoral collaboration involve the education and employment sectors. "Like the workplace, schools are an important environment for the prevention of mental ill-health. They need to be committed to improving or sustaining the mental and physical health of children. Mental health promotion in schools includes teaching about coping skills, improving self-esteem, learning to say 'no' to involvement in risk behaviours, and education about parenting and child-rearing skills" (WHO, 1998a).

Policy should incorporate a distribution of rights and responsibilities between the ministries of education and health.

Some examples of preventive and promotional activities in the field of mental health in schools are given below (Ministry of Health, Chile, 2000):

- respecting and practising human rights and solidarity;
- reinforcing citizenship participation, knowledge and skills for coping with personal and community life;
- developing self-esteem and emotional communication;
- developing social skills for communication, conflict resolution and gender equality;
- reinforcing skills for healthy lifestyles and self-care;
- preventing alcohol and drug abuse, violent behaviour and risky sex;
- detecting and supporting children with learning, emotional and behavioural problems;
- referral of children and adolescents with mental disorders to primary care and specialist services.

Collaboration with the employment sector is also vital. There is a growing awareness of the role of work in promoting mental health. Although it is difficult to quantify the impact of work alone on personal identity, self-esteem and social recognition, most experts agree that the workplace environment can have a significant influence on these variables.

Mental health policy should therefore consider the distribution of responsibilities between the ministry of labour and the ministry of health. The main strategies that have proved effective for increasing the level of mental health of employees are indicated below (WHO, 2000b):

- promotion of mental health in the workplace, including specific actions on job stress and the management of stress;
- protection of mental health in unemployed people by means of social and re-employment programmes;
- recognition of mental disorders in the workplace, including employee assistance programmes with early treatment and reintegration into the work environment;
- anti-discrimination provisions in legislation and the education of employers about the employment of people with mental disabilities;
- mechanisms for reintegrating people with serious mental disorders into work, including psychosocial rehabilitation, the development of work skills, supported employment and social enterprises.

Other sectors to consider for intersectoral collaboration are the stakeholders that were described in connection with the consultation process for developing mental health policy. (See examples in Box 2.)

Step 7. Identify the major roles and responsibilities of different sectors

In order for the areas for action to be carried out successfully it is essential that all the stakeholders responsible for carrying out the actions be identified and have a clear understanding of their roles and responsibilities. The stakeholders listed earlier are the main sectors to be considered when these roles and responsibilities are being determined.

- *Government agencies*: firstly, it is necessary to determine which government agency is going to be in charge of mental health policy. As mentioned earlier it is desirable for the head of government or the minister of health to have this responsibility.

The policy should define the roles of ministries along the following lines:

- *Health*: development of policy, regulation, evaluation, prevention and treatment;
- *Education*: promotional and preventive activities concerning mental health in schools;
- *Employment*: promotional and preventive activities in workplaces;
- *Social welfare*: rehabilitation, support for special needs and pension plans;
- *Housing*: supported housing for persons with disabilities;
- *Justice*: treatment and rehabilitation of persons in prisons, diversion of persons with mental disorders from the judicial system.

- *Academic institutions*: in countries with few human resources for mental health it is necessary for the ministry of health to establish regulations for training institutions. These should focus on training the type of workers required to address the mental health needs of the population, as identified by the mental health policy.

- *Professional associations*: policy can also determine the roles and responsibilities of these organizations. For example, in many places they play a significant role in regulating the practice of mental health workers by issuing licences and clinical and ethical guidelines.

There is a growing awareness of the role of work in promoting mental health.

The next step is to ident the roles and responsib of the different sectors involved in mental health

- *General health workers and mental health workers*: policy should determine the nature of the participation of workers in planning and should define workers' functions in the different services.

- *Consumer and family groups*: given the increasing level of organization that people with mental disorders and family groups are attaining in many countries, policy should cover their incorporation into the different levels of planning and evaluation processes. It is also necessary to determine which of their roles should be prioritized (e.g. advocacy, mutual help, providers of services).

- *Providers*: policy can define the financing and regulatory mechanisms to be used in the public and private sectors.

- *Nongovernmental organizations*: the role of nongovernmental organizations in the provision of mental health interventions requires definition in most countries or regions.

- *Traditional health workers*: traditional health workers are an available resource in many developing countries and can be included in policy if their ethical and technical responsibilities are well defined.

Key points: Areas for action and roles and responsibilities

-   Financing is a powerful tool for translating policy into reality and shaping mental health services and their outcomes.

-   Legislation can protect the rights of persons with mental disorders and contribute to promotion and prevention in the field of mental health.

-   Consumers, families and advocacy groups can have a significant role in the development of mental health policy.

-   Mental health services should be integrated into general health services, with community care and the movement of care away from psychiatric hospitals.

-   There is evidence of the effectiveness of a number of interventions relating to promotion, prevention, treatment and rehabilitation.

-   Directions for intersectoral collaboration, information systems, research, evaluation, quality improvement, essential drugs, and human resources and training should also be considered for inclusion in policies.

-   Roles and responsibilities: The areas for action should be allocated to government agencies, providers, consumers, nongovernmental organizations and health workers.

Examples of policies

Boxes 5 and 6 present summaries of mental health policies for two fictitious countries, one with a low level of resources for mental health and the other with a medium level of resources.

Box 5. Example of mental health policy for a country with a low level of resources*

Country A (10 000 000 inhabitants)
> Interviews with health workers and community leaders identified care for psychosis, epilepsy and intellectual disability as the main mental health needs of the population.
> At present only persons with severe psychosis and disruptive behaviour are admitted to the two mental hospitals, and outpatient treatment is limited to four cities (40% of the population) where specialists are available.
> The specialist level is formed by 20 psychiatrists, 30 psychologists and 80 psychiatric nurses (about 30-50% of their time is spent in private practice and teaching).

Mental health policy

1. Vision: Mental health care will deliver integrated, comprehensive community-based care that responds to the priority needs of psychosis, epilepsy and intellectual disability with an emphasis on prevention and early detection. Respect for the human rights of people with a mental disorder will guide service provision.

2. The following **values and principles** were supported by most stakeholders:

- Mental health is indivisible from general health: mental health care should be integrated into the primary care centres.
- Community care: persons with psychosis should be treated and cared for preferentially at home with the support of families and neighbours.
- Cultural relativism: traditional health workers should play a significant role.
- Accessibility: all people should have access to primary care, regardless of their economic status or geographical location.

3. Objectives: Each of the objectives selected had as a consideration the need to improve health, respond to people's expectations and provide financial protection

- To decrease the prevalence of common mental disorders and/or to reduce the level of disability caused by them.
- To protect the rights of persons with mental disorders.
- To increase the number of persons with mental disorders who are treated in primary care.

4. The following **areas for action** were set as priorities:

- **Legislation and human rights:** Because of the lack of protection for persons with severe mental disorders a new law addressing several rights needs to be formulated.
- **Financing:** Additional funds for mental health need to be allocated to primary health care in order to strengthen mental health interventions which are accessible to the community.
- **Research and evaluation:** Because of the lack of evidence about the prevention and treatment of mental disorders in primary care settings a pilot project needs to be set up to examine cost-effective strategies.
- **Organization of services:** Links between primary care teams and secondary services needs to be strengthened
- **Promotion, prevention, treatment and rehabilitation:** The following priorities were discussed:

- Prevention of brain damage through adequate prenatal care, safe delivery, immunization and the treatment of infectious diseases in early childhood;
- Treatment of persons with psychosis and epilepsy in primary care settings with the support of trained families and neighbours.
- **Human resources:** Because of the shortage of mental health professionals and the important role of traditional health workers in rural communities the following three priorities were discussed:
  - primary care workers need to be trained in mental health;
  - links need to be developed with traditional health workers;
  - nurses need to be trained in community psychiatry so that they can work in conjunction with primary care teams.

* the examples are not specific recommendations for action.

Box 6. Example of mental health policy for a country with a medium level of resources*

Country B (10 000 000 inhabitants)
> An epidemiological study of adults attending primary care centres showed the following prevalence rates: 18% for depression, 12% for anxiety disorders, 10% for alcohol abuse or dependence.
> Focus groups involving people from different backgrounds revealed needs for the care of adults with acute psychosis and suicidal behaviour and of children with learning and conduct problems.
> Some primary care centres deliver basic treatment for these mental disorders and one NGO has a programme on life skills and healthy school environments.
> Most of the mental health resources are concentrated in two cities, there being one large mental hospital and two inpatient units in general hospitals.
> There are 100 psychiatrists, 40 clinical psychologists, 250 psychiatric nurses and 40 occupational therapists working in mental health.

Mental health policy

Vision: Mental health of the population will be improved through mental health promotion in primary schools and ensuring the early treatment of mental disorders in primary care. Equity issues for people with severe mental disorders will be addressed throughout the health and social welfare systems.

Values and principles: In accordance with the vision, two lines of values and principles were agreed:

- *Psychological well-being*: Mental health promotion should be integrated into the actions of sectors other than health.
- *Indivisibility of mental health, general health and community care*: Mental health should be integrated into the general health system and community care should be developed with the participation of consumers and families.

Objectives: Each of the objectives selected had as a consideration the need to improve health, respond to people's expectations and provide financial protection

- To enhance life skills in school children, reduce the prevalence of depression and reduce complications of alcohol withdrawal.
- To improve consumers' satisfaction with mental health care.

- To achieve parity for mental health in social and private insurance.

The following **areas for action** were set as priorities:

- **Legislation and human rights:** Some mental health legislation has been developed. However, there is a need for social welfare support for people with mental disorders.
- **Financing:** Some funds were available for specialist mental health services. However, there was a need to improve funding for the integration of mental health services into primary care services.
- **Organization of services:** Screening and early treatment for depression, suicidal risk, psychosis and alcohol abuse needs to be implemented in primary care with the support of community mental health teams.
- **Essential drugs:** In order to develop these services in primary care centres the provision and use of essential psychotropic medicines needs to be ensured.
- **Intersectoral collaboration:** The need for a working alliance was discussed between the ministry of health and two other sectors:
  - *Social welfare:* In order to help people with schizophrenia to live in their communities;
  - *Education:* In order to implement mental health promotion activities in schools.
- **Advocacy:** The ministry of health has undertaken to achieve parity for mental health in public and private services and is discussing the need to involve consumers and families to participate in the planning and evaluation of mental health services.
- **Quality improvement:** The quality of treatment and care in primary health care needs to be improved drastically.

* the examples are not specific recommendations for action.

3. Developing a mental health plan

Once the mental health policy has been written (and, preferably, officially approved) it is necessary to formulate a plan for implementing the identified objectives by building on the process already established for policy development. The information about the population's needs, gathering evidence, consultation, negotiation, and exchange with other countries, which were required for the development of the policy, must be utilized and expanded upon in the formulation of a plan. Additional consultation and negotiation should be undertaken and any new information required should be collected. The next steps are to determine the strategies, activities, time frames, indicators and targets and the resources required for the plan.

Step 1. Determine the strategies and time frames

Strategies are the core aspect of a national or regional mental health plan. In many countries, indeed, plans are called "strategic plans" or simply "strategy". Strategies represent the lines of action which are thought to have the highest probability of successfully implementing the mental health policy in a given population. If properly designed in relation to the circumstances prevailing in a country or region, they allow rapid implementation of the mental health policy.

Strategies are the core aspect of a national or regional mental health plan.

Strategies are often formulated by conducting a SWOT analysis, i.e. by identifying the strengths, weaknesses, opportunities and threats associated with current mental health services and programmes.

- Some of the **strengths** of mental health services and programmes might be: motivation of human resources; collaboration of sectors other than health; successful outcomes with pilot projects; laws favouring mental health; family and consumer organizations; advocacy groups; the availability of some human resources (e.g. traditional health workers, nursing aides, mental health workers and psychologists).

- Some of the **weaknesses** of a mental health programme and services might be: scarce resources allocated to mental health; general health teams insufficiently trained in mental health; a fragmented health system with poor coordination between primary and specialist care; absence of an information system for mental health; insufficient activity for quality improvement.

The strengths and weaknesses of the present services and programmes are defined.

- Some of the **opportunities** for the development of mental health policy in a country might be: public awareness about poor living conditions or human rights violations affecting persons in psychiatric hospitals; a health reform process that is setting new priorities; public alarm about increasing violence or drug abuse.

- Some of the **threats** to the development of mental health policy in a country might be: strong stigma associated with mental disorders; a financial crisis and high unemployment rates; public opinion focused on subjects other than mental health.

On the basis of the SWOT analysis the following steps should be taken by the mental health division of the ministry of health.

Opportunities and threats the development of policy and plans defined.

1. List the main proposals in the mental health policy for each of the areas for action (Box 4). The list should also define which sectors would be in charge of each proposal in accordance with the policy's definition of roles and responsibilities.

2. Hold brainstorming sessions with experts in mental health and public health in order to define the principal strategies for implementing each of the proposals listed in the preceding step. This step requires the analysis of strengths, weaknesses, opportunities and threats, as described above.

3. Set priorities for the strategies elaborated in the second step, choosing two or three strategies for every area for action (Box 7). Once these are identified an additional priority-setting process can be conducted for the whole set of 20 to 30 strategies. A few can be selected as high priorities or all can be placed in order of priority. When carrying out this step it is advisable to consult and negotiate actively with representatives of the main stakeholders.

Box 7. Examples of strategies for a mental health plan

Areas for action	Strategies
1. Financing	- Any increment in mental health resources will be allocated to community services for persons with severe mental disorders. - A special fund will be created to support the incorporation of mental health interventions into primary health care. - Three priority mental health interventions will be included in the coverage of social health insurance.
2. Legislation and human rights	- A law will be drafted on the issue of involuntary admission. - A review board will be created to protect the rights of people with mental disorders. - A law on paid maternity leave, aimed at enhancing mother and child bonding, will be proposed to the legislature.
3. Organization of services	- Most persons with mental health disorders will be treated in primary care settings; fewer than 10 % will be referred to specialists. - Mental health specialists will meet primary care teams at least once a month to discuss cases and referral procedures. - Resources from psychiatric hospitals will be shifted towards general hospitals and community mental health teams.
4. Human resources and training	- A thorough review of the current supply of human resources for mental health will be undertaken and compared with estimates of the need for human resources. - Undergraduate training on the country's five mental health priorities will be introduced for all health professions. - Continuing professional development will be introduced for all qualified mental health staff. - A mental health in-service training course will be introduced for primary care workers.
5. Promotion, prevention, treatment and rehabilitation	- A suicide prevention programme will be implemented, including opportune treatment for depression and controls on guns and toxic substances. - An intellectual disability programme will be introduced, including prevention (iodine, counselling for pregnant women about alcohol), integration into regular

schools and vocational training.
- A school programme, including mental health promotion and early treatment of hyperkinetic disorders, will be established.

6. Essential drugs
- The provision of medication for depression, psychosis and epilepsy will be incorporated into primary care (two types of drugs for each condition).
- An atypical antipsychotic drug will be imported by a public institution and distributed at low cost.
- High-cost antidepressant medication will be dispensed through public insurance only under quality regulations.

7. Advocacy
- Technical support and funding will be given to consumer and family groups.
- A public campaign against stigma and discrimination will be developed in a demonstration area.
- Mental health workers will be trained in mental health advocacy.

8. Quality improvement
- Standards and accreditation will be developed for inpatient services, day hospitals, community mental health teams and halfway homes.
- Consumer and family groups will be educated on quality assurance and consulted about their assessment of services.
- Outcomes will be monitored in a programme for the treatment of depression in a primary care setting.

9. Information systems
- Mental health activities will be fully integrated into the health information system of the country concerned.
- Records of the numbers of mental health staff in each profession and psychiatric beds will be updated every year.
- The numbers of mental health patients and visits to primary health care will be registered every year during a period of two weeks.

10. Research and evaluation
- A demonstration area for national mental health policy will be evaluated for five years.
- Three professionals will be trained in the evaluation of mental health policy with the collaboration of a university in a developed country.
- 5% of health research funding will be devoted to mental health.

11. Intersectoral collaboration
- The prevention of alcohol and drug abuse among school children will be developed conjointly with the ministry of education.
- A programme for the management of work stress will be implemented in conjunction with the ministry of labour.
- A pilot project of supported employment for persons with schizophrenia will be developed with the ministry of labour.

Co-ordination of strategies is also required, for example one could imagine a country which has the discharge of patients from psychiatric institutions into well funded community care programmes, i.e. deinstitutionalization, as a major objective. This objective is consistent with improving health (through increased accessibility and quality of care), responding to people's expectations (most people prefer to be in the community) and providing financial protection (for example through providing disability grants). Implementation would then require co-ordinated strategies in and between a number of areas for action.

Implementation requires coordinated strategies in and between a number of areas for action.

Deinstitutionalization is clearly a major concern in the area of *organization of services*, but it requires cohesive and coherent responses involving other areas as well. For example discharging people into community care requires *financial* scheduling; *human resources* need to be trained and shifted; *advocacy* is required to change community attitudes; *essential drugs* need to be procured and distributed in the community; other government and non-governmental organizations such as housing, social services and labour need to become involved through *intersectoral collaboration*. In fact when fundamental mental health policy shifts such as deinstitutionalization occur, each and every area for action mentioned in Box 4 will need to be addressed.

Strategies under each area for action must be developed. For example:

Organization of services
- The least disabled patients should be prepared and be the first to be discharged from the psychiatric institutions
- Psycho-social rehabilitation programmes must be developed within the community;
- Day care centres must be set up for people who require close supervision

Financing
- Financial resources must be shifted from psychiatric hospitals to community programmes
- Additional finances must be obtained from donor agencies

Human resources and training
- General health practitioners must be trained to deal with mental health problems
- Professional mental health staff must provide a training and supervisory role in communities

Advocacy
- Mental health must be destigmatized in communities so that people's lives are improved through deinstitutionalization

Essential drug procurement and distribution
- All health clinics must have a prescribed range of psychotropic medication available

Intersectoral collaboration
- Community residential housing must be made available for people unable to be discharged into their family environment

In reality, in order to meet the goal of deinstitutionalization there would need to be more strategies under each area for action as well as under other areas.

The priority-setting described in the previous section should yield a list of strategies that are considered the most effective for the prevailing circumstances in the particular country or region. These should be implemented within a given period in accordance with a specified time frame. A convenient period for the implementation of a mental health plan can range from three to eight years.

However a time frame should also be defined for each strategy. It is necessary to state the intended year of commencement and the duration of each strategy. Some strategies need to keep functioning continuously and indefinitely. Others will operate only for a limited period. It frequently happens that strategies cannot be implemented in full as from the year of commencement because there are not enough resources or capacities. In these cases it is necessary to determine the extent to which the strategies will be implemented in the first year and how much will be added every subsequent year.

Time frames are defined for each strategy with dates of commencement and duration.

Box 8. Example of a time frame for a mental health plan

	Year 1	Year 2	Year 3	...etc.
Degree of implementation of strategies every year				
Strategy 1	100%	To continue indefinitely		
Strategy 2			100%	End
Strategy 3	50%	100%		End
Strategy 4			50%	100%
Strategy 5	33%	66%	100%	To continue
...etc.				

Box 8 shows how to write a time frame for a national or regional mental health plan. Strategy 1 involves implementation from the first year and indefinite maintenance, probably until the next plan is developed. Strategy 2 can be utilized later and for a limited period; this type of strategy generally involves high capital expenditure. Strategy 3 is also applied for a limited time but it begins on a partial basis and reaches full implementation after two or three years. Strategy 4 involves late and partial introduction and has to be sustained indefinitely. Strategy 5 starts gradually at the beginning of the plan and it too has to be sustained indefinitely.

Notwithstanding the determination of strategies and time-frames described, the plan is incomplete until the details of how it will be implemented are drawn up. It is necessary to have targets, with indicators, which will show whether the strategies have been realized or not. It is important too to list all the activities and the costs and resources that are required. The specific time frames must also be determined. Steps 2-4 address these issues. It should be noted, however, that these steps will not necessarily happen consecutively and in fact will often need to be planned interdependently and simultaneously. For example targets, indicators and activities are all dependent on availability of resources while activities will influence targets and indicators.

The plan is incomplete until the details of how it will be implemented are drawn up.

Step 2. Set Indicators and targets

Once the strategies have been determined, they must be broken down into specific targets and *indicators* drawn up to later assess whether the plan has been effective or not.

Strategies should have clear targets of what must be achieved and, as already mentioned, a time frame in which to achieve them. It must be clear how the individual activities will contribute to the target.

Strategies should have targets of what must be achieved and a time frame in which to achieve them.

The first strategy under *organization of services* illustrates this (see Box 9). If the least disabled patients must be prepared and discharged from the psychiatric institutions, a target of how many patients this would involve must be set. If the target was for 20% of all institutionalized patients to be discharged within one year, this target would then need to be aligned with targets for other strategies, for example, the number of community based rehabilitation programmes that will need to be set up and where; which staff will be trained and placed in the community to meet the needs of these discharged patients; how much money will be shifted from the hospital to "follow" these patients and so on. This alignment is very important to ensure that activities are not undertaken merely to meet isolated targets. For example while a target of 20% discharges may be relatively easy to meet by simply releasing patients, unless other targets are reached simultaneously, these patients may land in the streets without receiving any services at all.

Strategies must be concrete, feasible and measurable. Planners must thus develop "indicators" to assess whether the strategy has been realized or not. This often requires collection of information or data at the time that the strategy is devised. For example if 20% of the least disabled patients are going to be discharged from psychiatric hospitals, it is necessary for the planner to know firstly how many people are currently in hospitals and secondly the levels of disability of all these patients. Only if such information is available at the beginning of the plan, is it possible to measure whether the target has been reached or not at the end of the time period.

Planners must develop "indicators" to assess whether the strategy has been realized or not.

While numbers or percentages are often good indicators to use, not all outcomes can be measured in this way. For example an indicator for decreased stigmatization may be measured in terms of changed community attitudes which may be conducted through a specifically designed attitudinal survey or a focus group discussion. Moreover, there may be more than one indicator for a strategy.

Step 3. Determine the major activities

Some planning questions that can be addressed through having a comprehensive plan are:

- What "activities" are necessary to implement a particular strategy?
- Who will take responsibility for each activity?
- How long will each activity take?
- Which activities can be done simultaneously and which can only follow the completion of another activity?
- What are the outputs expected from each activity?
- What are the potential obstacles or delays that could inhibit the realization of each activity and can steps be taken to obviate these?

While this may seem a complex set of issues, it need not be. By drawing up simple tables for each strategy, it is relatively easy to cover all these questions (See Box 9). This process also enables planners to bring together the objectives previously identified, as well as various areas of action, into a single planning framework.

There are two important reasons to list activities in some detail. Most importantly it ensures that important steps are not missed out and each component necessary to meet the objective is carefully thought through. Secondly, it is not trivial to mark one's successes. If one sets only activities that are large and very difficult to achieve, it is difficult to note progress and to feel that the large objective is being reached. This can be highly demotivating. Activities should be set within time frames, and if these time frames are realistic and in fact reached, it is possible to be constantly reinforced by one's own achievements.

As shown in Box 9, by dividing the year into months (or quarters if preferable), a planner can systematically arrange each activity into a realistic timetable. By designing a plan on a monthly or other periodic basis it is possible to clearly determine what activity has to follow the completion of another activity and also what can or should be done simultaneously. By listing the time related activities and comparing across the total objectives, it is possible to assess whether the year's plan is feasible and realistic, but also ensure that activities are spread across the year. For example a systematic method helps to ensure that many highly time consuming activities are not planned for the same

A list of activities must be drawn up for each strategy.

Box 9 Three strategies derived from the objective of deinstitutionalization are presented.

Examples are taken from *Organization of Services*, *Human Resources and Financing*. Similar detailed plans would need to be drawn up for each strategy in each area for action. This plan covers a one year period.

Objective: Reducing the number of people in psychiatric institutions and increasing the number of people receiving community care

Area for action: Organization of Services
Strategy 1: The least disabled patients should be prepared and discharged from the psychiatric institutions
Targets: 20% of the least disabled patients will have been prepared and discharged
Indicator: The proportion of patients discharged from psychiatric institutions

Activity	Jan	Feb	Mar	Apr	May	Jun	Jul	Aug	Sep	Oct	Nov	Dec	Responsible person	Output	Potential obstacles
Assess level of disability of each hospitalized patient from study conducted	●	●											District mental health managers Provincial health department	20% of least disabled patients identified	Instruments used to assess disability are not culturally appropriate
Assess home circumstance of the least disabled 20%		●	●										District mental health managers	Home visits conducted	Family members don't want patients back and are uncooperative
Determine which of these patients can be discharged to families and who will require housing			●	●									District mental health managers	List of who will be discharged to families and who will require accommodation	Very few patients able to be returned to their families
Conduct psycho-social discharge programme			●	●	●	●	●	●					Hospital managers	Programme completed for each patient	Hospital staff have no skills in preparing people for discharge
Liaise with Ministry of Housing for accommodation to be made available				●	●								National Ministry of Health, Ministry of Housing	Agreement reached with Ministry of Housing	Ministry of Housing not able to provide housing for the mentally disabled
Liaise with NGO for setting up day care					●	●							District mental health managers	Agreement reached with NGOs for day care centres	No NGOs available with knowledge of how to run day care centres
Discharge patients into organized community services							●	●	●	●	●		Hospital managers in conjunction with district mental health managers	Patients discharged into community care programmes	Community programmes not available to discharge patients from hospital and no funds shifted

Objective: Reducing the number of people in psychiatric institutions and increasing the number of people receiving community care

Strategy 1: General health practitioners must deal with people with mental health problems
Targets: 20 community based doctors and 50 nurses trained to provide mental health care as part of general health care
Indicator: Number of community based doctors and nurses trained

Activity	Jan	Feb	Mar	Apr	May	Jun	Jul	Aug	Sep	Oct	Nov	Dec	Responsible person	Output	Potential obstacles
Meeting to be held with district health managers in 5 disctricts		●											National Ministry (A. Other)	Objectives agreed with managers	Mental health may not be prioritized by district managers
District managers to identify 4 doctors and 10 nurses per district for training		●											District Managers (Put names)	Doctors and nurses to be trained identified	Doctors and nurses may not be available for mental health training and may not want to undertake mental health work
Universities and colleges to be contacted to conduct the training		●											Provincial Authorities (Put names)	Agreement reached on responsibility for training and time frames	Academics may be involved with their own teaching and research activities
Training to take place in each district				●	●	●	●	●					Universities/ Colleges	Training completed in time frames	Insufficient resources have been made available in the district for in-service training
Support and supervision to be provided to trained practitioners					●	●	●	●	●	●	●	●	Psychiatrist and psychiatric nurses at district level	A record of each supervision and support recorded	Transport to travel within the district is not available therefore on the job supervision is not provided
Plan survey to assess which patients are receiving care through integrated mental health services with researcher						●	●						National Ministry with research body	Survey agreed to and planned	Resources to carry out evaluation are not available
Start monitoring and evaluation										●	●		Research body	Survey started	District managers do not allow the researchers access to records

53

Objective: Reducing the number of people in psychiatric institutions and increasing the number of people receiving community care

Area for action: Financing
Strategy 1: Financial resources must be shifted from psychiatric hospitals to community programmes
Targets: Transfer of proportionate resources as calculated in activities one and two
Indicators: Proportionate resources available in the community for mental health care

Activity	Jan	Feb	Mar	Apr	May	Jun	Jul	Aug	Sep	Oct	Nov	Dec	Responsible person	Output	Potential obstacles
Calculate the cost per patient day in institutional care	●	●											Financial section within Ministry of Health	Costs available	Costs not available
Calculate the marginal savings to hospitals by having 20% fewer patients		●	●	●									Financial section within Ministry of Health	Costing done	Disagreements around how much money can be saved by discharging 20% of patients
Transfer the saved finances from the hospital to the community when patients are discharged								●	●	●	●	●	Financial section within Ministry of Health	Finances transferred	Difficulties with transferring finances from one budget item to another

Examples of plans

Boxes 10 and 11 present examples of priority strategies in the mental health plans of the two fictitious countries described in Boxes 5 and 6.

Box 10. Examples of priority strategies in the mental health plan of a country with a low level of resources*

Country A (same as in Box 5)

Area for action: Legislation and human rights
Strategy: Formulating a mental health law to protect the rights of persons with mental disorders
Target: A new mental health law which protects the rights of persons with mental disorders within two years. Indicator: A new mental health law enacted.
Activities (within first year):
- Review the current law against international human rights instruments
- Examine laws from other countries with similar social and cultural situations
- Organize meetings with key stakeholders to discuss the content of legislation
- Draft first version of legislation and circulate it for comment

Area for action: Financing
Strategy: The allocation of funds to strengthen preventive and curative mental health interventions in primary care settings
Target: An additional 30% of funds from the current funding allocation to go to preventive and curative mental health interventions in primary care
Indicator: Proportion of funds allocated to preventive and curative mental health interventions in primary care
Activities:
- Lobby within the Ministry of Health for equity between physical and mental health services
- Collect information from other countries on the cost benefit of a programme to prevent a particular mental health problem
- Prepare a funding application to submit to chosen donor organizations

Area for action: Research and evaluation
Strategy: A pilot project for the prevention and treatment of mental disorders in primary care to be funded by and evaluated in collaboration with an international agency
Target: Pilot project completed and evaluated
Indicator: Research results of a pilot project for the prevention and treatment of mental disorders in primary care
Activities:
- Identify the specific problem and the research required to answer the problem
- Get agreement from skilled researchers both inside the country and internationally on the methodology to be used and their agreement to carry out the research
- Prepare the funding application for the research
- Monitor progress of research and intervene to get it on track if necessary
- Ensure research results are written into a report with recommendations

Area for action: Organization of services.
Strategy: Mental health specialists (including psychiatrists, psychologists and psychiatric nurses) will provide supervision and receive referrals from primary care workers.
Target: 75% of all mental health specialists providing supervision and receiving referrals from primary care workers

Indicator: Percentage of mental health specialists providing supervision and receiving referrals from primary care workers

Activities:

- Negotiate with mental health specialists to provide supervision and be available for referral
- Arrange a transportation system to allow the agreed upon plan to be implemented

Area for action: Promotion, prevention, treatment and rehabilitation.

Strategy: A primary health care programme on psychosis and epilepsy involving nurses.

Target: 50% of nurses in primary care able to deliver antipsychotic and antiepileptic medication

Indicator: Percentage of nurses in primary care able to deliver antipsychotic and antiepileptic medication

Activities:

- Meet with nurses to explain the policy and discuss difficulties they may have with the policy
- Organize training with a training institution and the regional health managers
- Training of health workers to be conducted

Area for action: Human resources and training

Strategy: A training programme for community psychiatric nurses

Target: 3 psychiatric nurses per million population within a year and twenty per million within ten years

Indicator: Number of psychiatric nurses per million population

Activities:

- Start training of psychiatric nurses in newly opened nursing school
- Ensure that curriculum covers all the needs of nurses within a primary care situation

* the examples are not specific recommendations for action.

Box 11. Examples of priority strategies in the mental health plan of a country with a medium level of resources*

Country B (same as in Box 6)

Area for action: Legislation and human rights.

Strategy: The provision of a disability pension for people with schizophrenia.

Target: 50% of people diagnosed with schizophrenia and disabled to the extent of being unable to be employed on the open market receiving disability grants within three years.

Indicator: Percentage of people diagnosed with schizophrenia and disabled to the extent of being unable to be employed on the open market receiving disability grants.

Activities:

- Develop an assessment tool to determine who is eligible for a disability grant
- Publicize the availability of grants through health facilities and the media
- Set up systems for people with schizophrenia to be assessed for eligibility for a disability grant
- Set up systems for the payment of disability grants in collaboration with the Departments of Welfare and Finance
- Begin assessments in ten pilot areas

Area for action: Financing

Strategy: Matching the resources that were recycled locally for mental health at primary care centres with new funding

Target: New funding equal to one half of locally recycled funds within one year and equal funding within two years

Indicator: Amount of new funding for mental health services

Activities:

- Hold negotiations with the Department of Finance to secure funding within the targeted period
- Have meetings with district health officials to ensure that the resources allocated are utilized for mental health and not for any other identified priority
- Set of a monitoring system to assess who is benefiting from the additional funding

Area for action: Organization of services

Strategy: The reutilization of resources from the mental hospital in order to strengthen community programmes

Target: 10% of all capital expenditure, human resources and consumables to be allocated to primary care services within year one; 40% within year two and 70% within year three

Indicator: Percentage of expenditure, human resources and consumables to be allocated to primary care services

Activities:

- Hold discussions with labour unions, psychiatric hospital authorities, drug distribution organizations and consumer and family groups regarding the intended changes
- Create posts within primary care settings to deal with the additional load at this level
- Train and prepare staff for implementation of this strategy
- Prepare patients for discharge and discharge them at the appropriate time

Area for action: Essential drugs

Strategy: Antidepressant, antipsychotic and antianxiety medication to be available within regional and district health services

Target: Specific drugs to treat depression, psychosis and anxiety to be available in 50% of health facilities at regional level and 30% at primary level within year one and 80% and 50% respectively in year two

Indicator: Availability of specific drugs to treat depression, psychosis and anxiety in health facilities at regional and primary care levels

Activities:

- Call a meeting of experts in psychiatric care (at different levels of health care), together with personnel responsible for drug procurement, finances and consumer representatives to draw up a list of essential drugs to be available at the regional and district levels.
- Circulate the list and incorporate comments
- Hold planning meetings with managers of primary care services at primary and district levels to arrange for the implementation of the plan
- Monitor the availability of drugs at the services chosen to initially implement the plan and adapt the plan accordingly

Area for action: Intersectoral collaboration

Strategy: Partner the ministry of education in implementing a life skills intervention in public schools

Target: 50% coverage within year three and 100% coverage of all public schools within six years

Indicator: Percentage of public schools having life skills intervention

Activities:

- Meet with the department of education to agree on a vision and a plan for life skills education in schools
- Tender out the development of the intervention to an appropriate team of local experts

- Test the intervention in specified pilot schools and adapt the programme
- Ensure that the department of education includes the intervention in the curriculum of the targeted schools within a stepped process of implementation

Area for action: Advocacy
Strategy: People with mental disorders and their families should participate in the planning and evaluation of mental health services
Target: Full participation of consumer and family groups in planning and implementation of services within all health districts, primary care centres and mental health facilities within 4 years. 35% coverage to be achieved within two years
Indicator: Percentage of facilities where mental health planning and evaluation is undertaken with full participation of consumers and family members
Activities:
- Consult with consumer and family representatives at national level and get consensus on the plan. Request the representatives to disseminate the plan to branches at local levels
- Identify areas where there is strong local consumer and family participation and involve them in the process of planning and evaluation of services
- Train more consumers to enable them to participate in planning and evaluation
- Roll out the involvement of consumers and families taking into account difficulties experienced and lessons learnt

Area for action: Quality improvement
Strategy: Clinical guidelines, standards and an accreditation system for mental health will be developed for primary care centres conjointly with professional associations in the health field
Target: Clinical guidelines for identified conditions available within one year and standards and an accreditation system available within two years
Indicator: Clinical guidelines for identified conditions, standards, and an accreditation system available
Activities:
- Meet with relevant professional associations and formulate a plan for the development of clinical guidelines, standards and an accreditation system for primary care
- Appoint a team of experts from the ministry and the professional associations to formulate drafts based on current evidence based practices
- Circulate and incorporate comments on the drafts
- Follow country procedures for obtaining legal recognition for the accreditation system

* the examples are not specific recommendations for action.

4. Developing a mental health programme

Mental health *policy* focuses on values, principles and objectives. A plan is a detailed scheme, which allows for the implementation of the *policy*. Through the policy and plan a country is able to not only put mental health onto a well thought through and designed trajectory, but to put in place the mechanisms for realizing the policy goals. The plan formalizes the policy into a set of clear strategic and operational components, which assist countries in reaching their goals. However, in addition to these plans it is often advantageous to introduce targeted *programmes* into mental health. It is advisable for teams or individuals making mental health plans, including people within the Ministry of Health, to provide "spaces" within their own work (and within the work of the people who implement the services) for programmes to be included and implemented.

There are many reasons why, at different points, particular priorities come to the fore and have to be dealt with. These should not be seen as distractions or disruptions to achieving the longer term mental health goals, or deflections from previous prioritization processes, but as an integral part of providing mental health services.

Each country will have unique reasons why a programme may need to be implemented at a particular time. Some examples are:

- The cabinet decides that violence against women is an immediate national priority and that all departments must introduce programmes for prevention of violence and caring for victims. A programme for mental health care and rehabilitation must therefore be set up.
- A research project carried out by a well-known academic shows that Fetal Alcohol Syndrome is at unprecedented levels within a country. The Minister of Health responds by saying that programmes for the prevention of alcohol amongst pregnant women would be undertaken.
- A war breaks out in a neighbouring country. Tens of thousands of refugees, mostly women and children, have fled across the border. Many are suffering from severe psychological distress while others with chronic mental disorder no longer have access to medication. A programme is urgently needed.
- The Department of Corrections has signed an international agreement following which they are no longer permitted to hold people with mental disorder in prisons. They request the Department of Health to assist in providing secure mental health facilities.
- The World Health Organization negotiates to have mental health as the theme for World Health Day. Countries are requested to organize activities to reduce stigma and promote mental health.
- An international campaign is launched to treat epilepsy. Your country agrees to participate.
- The Minister of Health is lobbied by a consumer group for an amendment to one section of the mental health legislation. The minister agrees to investigate this fully.

A programme is often a shorter-term initiative than a policy or plan. However, this does not imply that programmes should not undergo thorough planning.

Steps outlined in the process of developing policy and plans are also relevant for programmes. As the details of these steps have already been outlined previously they are not repeated here. However, those involved in developing programmes should go through the following processes:

- Determine strategies and time frames based on research and information collected.

In addition to plans it is often advantageous to introduce targeted programmes into mental health.

At different points, particular priorities come to the fore and have to be dealt with.

A programme is a shorter-term initiative than a policy or plan, nonetheless it should undergo thorough planning.

- Set indicators and targets
- Determine the major activities and how and by whom these will be implemented
- Determine the costs and available resources and orientate the programme accordingly
- Set up monitoring and evaluation processes

Key points: Developing a mental health programme

- Programmes are often shorter term initiatives aimed at realizing specific identified goals.

- Mental health planners should accommodate programmes into their workplan in conjunction with longer term policies and plans.

- Programmes should follow similar steps to the development of plans. For example programmes should be evidence based, time frames must be set, major activities must be determined, targets and indicators must be set, costs, resources and responsible agents must be determined and every programme must be carefully monitored and evaluated.

5. Implementation issues for policy, plans and programmes

A mental health policy can be implemented through the priority strategies identified by the plan and the priority interventions identified by the plan/programme. The implementation of these strategies and interventions requires several actions (Fig. 1). The main actions relate to: the dissemination of the policy; political support and funding; -supportive organization; demonstration areas; the empowerment of providers; intersectoral coordination; interaction between the ministry of health and several stakeholders (including the allocation of funds, management, purchasing of services and regulation).

Step 1. Disseminate the policy

Once the mental health policy and plan have been formulated it is important that the ministry of health **disseminate and communicate the policy** to the health district offices and other partner agencies, targeting key individuals. Many policies fail simply because they are poorly communicated. It is a specific function of the mental health professionals in the ministry of health and the health districts to disseminate the new policy widely to all the stakeholders. Some ways of facilitating this process are suggested below.

> Organize a public event with the media at which the ministry of health or another government body officially introduces the new policy, plans and programmes.
> Print booklets on the policy, plans and programmes and distribute them to stakeholders.
> Print and distribute posters and leaflets which indicate the main ideas of the policy.
> Hold meetings with health teams, consumers, families, advocacy groups and other stakeholders in order to analyse the policy, plans and programmes.
> Organize national and international seminars to discuss mental health policies.
> Recruit and support consumer, family and other advocacy groups that will disseminate the policy.

The ministry of health and the health districts should disseminate the policy to stakeholders.

Step 2. Generate political support and funding

After a policy has been written, active stakeholder participation and communication activities should be initiated. These activities should last for a few months in order to ensure that enough **political support and funding** are given for implementation. In many instances, especially in developing countries, excellent written policies are not implemented or are only partially implemented because resources are insufficient.

Political support and funding must be given for the implementation of the policy.

It is essential to have well-placed persons who can advocate the policy at the highest levels of government and in key agencies. It is desirable for the population to be so well informed that it will not be satisfied unless mental health is pushed up the government agenda to meet their needs and demands. This rarely happens by chance.

The mental health professionals in the ministry of health should become involved in interviews and meetings with the authorities of their own ministry and other ministries, such as those of social welfare, employment/labour, education, justice, environment, housing, finance and trade and industry. They should also hold interviews and meetings with representatives of other institutions, such as parliament, the courts of justice, the police, local government and municipalities.

The authorities should be made aware that mental disorders represent a significant proportion of the burden of disease and that they generate important needs and demands.

The goal of these actions is to demonstrate the importance of mental health. The authorities should be made aware that mental disorders represent a significant proportion of the burden of disease (DALYs) and that they generate important needs and demands. They should appreciate that there are effective strategies and that all sectors can contribute towards improving the mental health of the population.

Step 3. Develop supportive organization

The implementation of mental health policy requires a competent group of professionals with expertise in both public health and mental health. This group should be responsible for managing plans and programmes, ensuring that the population can access mental health interventions of high quality which are responsive to expressed needs. This group should also be responsible for facilitating the active participation of people with mental disorders and their families in all the components of the mental health network, including collaborative intersectoral actions.

The organization supporting mental health policy should be present in all the administrative and geographical divisions of the country or region's health system (Asioli, 2000). The following levels, which may require adaptation to the circumstances in each country or region, may be considered.

> Ministry of health
In several countries it has proved very useful to have a multidisciplinary team in charge of national or regional mental health policy, plans and programmes. The size of the team will vary, of course, with that of the country or region, the resources available and the priority given to mental health, e.g. from two part-time persons in small countries or regions with few resources for mental health to more than 10 full-time people in larger countries or regions with more resources. The types of professionals to be considered include psychiatrists, public health physicians, psychologists, psychiatric nurses, social workers and occupational therapists.

The main functions of this team are to develop, manage, monitor and evaluate the policy, plans and programmes. The team also has to support and coordinate with consumer and family groups and to conduct advocacy initiatives. (For more details see Annex 3.)

> Health district
A mental health professional or, preferably, a multidisciplinary team similar to the one in the ministry of health, is required in each of the areas of the country or region in order to implement a local mental health plan or programme. The size of these teams will vary with the size of the health district. Their functions are described in Annex 3.

> Community mental health teams
It is highly recommended that each community mental health team (or comparable group involved in specialized mental health care) should have a coordinator. This person should devote a few hours a week, in addition to her or his regular promotional, preventive and clinical activities, to public health and management work. He or she will be responsible for liaising with the health district and attending coordination meetings. The functions of this professional include coordinating the activities of the members of the team, ensuring that guidelines are used, defining referral procedures and liaising with other health facilities and sectors (Annex 3).

> Primary health care teams
As with the community mental health teams it is advisable for each primary care facility or team to have a mental health coordinator. This person should devote a few hours each week to public health and management work. He or she will be responsible for liaison with the coordinator of the community mental health team and will attend coordination meetings (Annex 3).

The implementation of mental health policy req a competent group of professionals with exper in both public health an mental health.

A multidisciplinary team should be in charg of the policy, plan and programme at the level of the ministry of health.

A multidisciplinary team should be in charge of p plans and programmes at the level of the health district.

A coordinator is needed in each community mental health team.

A mental health coordina is needed in each primar health care team.

Step 4. Set up pilot projects in demonstration areas

It is recommended that the ministry of health establish pilot projects in (a) **demonstration area(s)** where policy, plans and programmes can be implemented more rapidly and evaluated more thoroughly than elsewhere in the country. The demonstration area can be a geographical region or a sector of a large city, provided that it is representative of the majority of the country's population. The knowledge that may be gained from a demonstration area is vital for the success of the policy and plan in the whole country.

Pilot projects test whether implementation is possible under the financial restrictions and usual conditions of the country's health system. This can facilitate the process of application on a larger scale subsequently.

One example of a pilot project that may have a strong influence in the formulation of a mental health policy is the transformation of a psychiatric hospital into a network of community facilities and services. Many mental health professionals have received all their training and have spent all their professional lives in psychiatric hospitals. It may be very difficult for them to accept that the same or better clinical outcomes are attainable in the community for people with serious mental disorders.

Another kind of pilot experience with a significant potential influence on policy formulation is that of the introduction of psychiatric beds into a general hospital. In many countries, physicians and general health professionals resist this development. They feel uncomfortable when they are near people undergoing psychotic episodes or expressing suicidal ideas. A pilot project can be a useful means of assessing these professional attitudes and the potential for change.

A pilot project is also helpful for orienting and informing mental health professionals in the health districts, where they can learn how to implement the policy in their own localities. It also serves as a training centre, where health staff from other districts can learn about new public health, promotive, preventive and clinical skills.

The knowledge that may be gained from a demonstration area is vital for the success of the policy in the whole country.

Key points: Implementing the basic support for the policy

- Policy should be disseminated to all stakeholders through public events, meetings, seminars and publications.

- Advocacy activities should be conducted in order to build political support and funding for the implementation of the policy.

- A supporting organization should be developed, with professionals in charge of the policy in every administrative division.

- Pilot projects can help with orienting the implementation of the policy and can serve as a training centre.

Step 5. Empower mental health providers

Providers in a health system are teams or institutions that deliver health interventions to the population. Both general health providers and specialist mental health providers deliver mental health interventions. Moreover, some institutions outside the health sector provide interventions. It is essential for the professionals in charge of mental health in the ministry of health to know how the different types of providers function in the country and how they relate to each other within the mental health system. This knowledge

The ministry of health needs to know how the different types of providers function in order that resources can be used efficiently.

makes it possible to use existing resources more efficiently and to deliver better mental health interventions.

The characteristics of providers may have a strong influence on the way that mental health interventions are delivered to the population. The best providers are **small multidisciplinary teams**, comprising persons from different fields who combine their skills and use their collective wisdom to deal with the complexities of the population's mental health. These multidisciplinary teams can be both at the primary care level and the specialized mental health level.

However, such providers are not always available, even in developed countries, because of insufficient resources or inadequate organization of the health system. Consequently, **individuals** (e.g. traditional health workers, family physicians, psychiatrists) deliver most mental health interventions in many countries. These individuals are disadvantaged by working in isolation from other professionals and by not having all the necessary skills for responding to the varying mental health needs of the populations concerned. They may also be comparatively reluctant to incorporate new interventions proposed in national or regional plans and programmes or to accept regulations from the ministry of health.

Institutions (e.g. hospitals, outpatient clinics), on the other hand, have different problems as providers. They tend to be too large, in spite of their economies of scale, and too remote from the people. Sometimes they become bureaucratic, authoritarian and impersonal. Institutionalization may develop, even when persons are treated on an ambulatory basis.

Six types of health providers are described below with specific reference to their empowerment. At present, most countries have a mixture of these types of providers.

5.5.1 Public mental health providers

Public mental health providers are organized in national or regional health services, and the State is the owner of the health facilities (hospitals and ambulatory clinics). In this system it is relatively easy to develop a national mental health policy because there is direct control over the services. The services are usually free but access may be limited because of shortages of resources.

One of the potential shortcomings of the public system is its vulnerability to the interests of the providers. This may make it rigid, inefficient, of low quality and unresponsive to the needs and expectations of populations (WHO, 2000a). In countries where public providers play a major role in the delivery of mental health interventions the ministry of health should contemplate strategies for empowering them through incentives.

Some examples of **incentives** for empowering public mental health providers are given below. (See the module *Mental Health Financing*.)

> **Autonomy:** The decentralization of the power structure and decision-making processes from the ministry of health to the health districts and from them to health facilities and teams.

> **Accountability:** The establishment of a contractual relationship between the ministry of health and the health districts and between them and the health facilities and teams. The contracts should have mutually agreed goals and economic incentives for their achievement.

> **Market exposure:** Instead of distributing all the resources through a direct budget allocation to health facilities and teams the ministry of health can introduce competition among them for prepaid revenues.

> **Financial responsibility:** The ministry of health may wish to relinquish total control of health finances in order that health facilities and teams assume responsibility for losses and profits.

5.5.2 Private mental health providers

Private mental health providers tend to function in response to market conditions. As a result it is more difficult for professionals at the ministry of health to involve them in policy, plans and programmes that set priorities and interventions. These providers have the advantage of being more open to innovations and more flexible in responding to the needs and expectations of populations. They usually function in response to incentives that the public providers lack.

On the other hand, private providers have the major disadvantage of exposing individuals to the financial risks of serious and long-lasting mental disorders. Often their treatments are not fully covered by insurance, and out-of-pocket payments may only be affordable to rich people. Their work is market-driven and can become dispersed. There is also the possibility of creating perverse incentives that induce providers to take advantage of people with mental disability.

Several problems can arise where substantial private provision exists and is paid for out-of-pocket in the absence of public funding and regulation. For instance, the poor may consume large amounts of low-quality mental health care from unregulated private mental health care providers such as drug sellers, traditional healers and unqualified therapists (WHO, 2001a).

In countries and regions where private providers play a significant role in the delivery of mental health services the ministry of health should consider their active participation in the formulation and implementation of policy, plans and programmes. Some strategies for empowering private providers and facilitating their participation are indicated below:

There are several strategies for empowering private providers and facilitating their participation.

> **Contractual relationship:** Contracts are established between the ministry of health or health districts and private providers for the delivery of some of the prioritized mental health interventions. This relationship should rely on professional reputation and a strong sense of commitment and responsibility rather than on close supervision and control. Depending on the characteristics of the health system, some countries can contract mainly with private providers for the delivery of interventions defined in their mental health plans/programmes. In other instances these providers will be the preferential providers for only some specific interventions.

> **Pooling of resources:** Pooling (from tax, social insurance or prepayment) can be done by the ministry of health, other public institutions and private insurance. The mental health professionals in the ministry of health should ensure that priority interventions are included in these service arrangements with private providers.

> **Regulation:** The mechanisms that have been used more extensively are guidelines, standards and accreditation. Private providers should be regulated by these mechanisms and the same standards should be applied as for public providers. Information on the guidelines, standards and accreditation should be disseminated to the general population so that proper choices can be made when these providers are being used.

> **Quality improvement:** Private providers need not only be passive recipients of regulation but should also be actively committed to the pursuit of improvements in the quality of their work. They can make a valuable contribution to the implementation of policy, plans

and programmes by defining quality procedures and standards and by carrying out accreditation through nongovernmental organizations that represent their interests.

5.5.3 Traditional health workers

Traditional medicine plays an important role in the promotional, preventive and curative aspects of health for a large percentage of the population, especially in developing countries. For this reason, traditional health workers should be incorporated as a resource for primary care whenever possible and appropriate. Some options whereby mental health professionals in the ministry of health might empower traditional healers are listed below:

- establishing links with a view to working cooperatively;
- teaching mental health practices to traditional healers in order to improve competencies;
- accreditation for the regulation of practice;
- referral and counter-referral systems for people with mental disorders (for example, traditional healers can deal with mild and moderate emotional conditions and can refer epilepsy and psychosis to formal health care providers);
- incorporating traditional healers into primary care or mental health facilities as translators (language and culture) and/or providers of some interventions.

Traditional health worke could be incorporated a a resource for primary health care.

5.5.4 Mutual aid groups

These groups encourage people with a problem to take control over the circumstances of their lives. Self-help is founded on the principle that people with the same disability have something to offer each other which cannot be provided by professionals (Goering, 1997). There are several alternative ways in which mental health professionals in health ministries can work with these groups:

- public education on the availability and benefits of mutual aid;
- training on mutual aid in the regular curricula of health and mental health managers and professionals;
- joint meetings of mental health professionals and representatives of mutual aid groups;
- steps to attract and train leaders of the mutual aid movement;
- research support for mutual aid.

People with the same disability have somethin to offer each other whic. cannot be provided by professionals.

5.5.5 Nongovernmental, voluntary and charitable organizations

In most countries there are various non-profit organizations that provide interventions aimed at helping people to improve their mental health. They have the advantages of grass-roots vitality, closeness to people, freedom to take individual initiatives, and opportunities for participation in and the humanization of mental health care (WHO, 1994). However, they also require delimitation of their scope of action and authority to oversee the accountability of funds and prevent certain difficulties that have arisen.

Mental health professionals in the ministry of health might consider the following options for empowering NGOs and incorporating them into the implementation of policy:

- funding mechanisms for professional NGOs on a contractual basis with a view to fostering their development;
- joint research aimed at introducing innovative mental health interventions into the country concerned;
- contracts for the provision of interventions to vulnerable populations (particularly those with whom NGOs have good relationships and experience),

NGOs have the advantag of grass-roots vitality, closeness to people and freedom to take individu. initiatives.

including the poor, children from disrupted homes, abused women, victims of violence, migrants, indigenous ethnic minorities and persons with disabilities.

5.5.6 Mental health consumers and families as providers

The term "consumer" applies to people who have or have had a mental disorder and have also been involved in the health care system. (See the module *Advocacy for Mental Health* for more details about consumers.) A health consumer may also be a person (1) willing to be involved in the planning, development, management and evaluation of services, and (2) willing to be consulted about the care, support and treatment that he or she will receive (WHO, 1989). Moreover, the families of people with mental disorders have played a significant role in the development of mental health systems in many countries.

The mental health professionals in charge of mental health in ministries of health should be in touch with the consumer and family movements of their countries or regions, and there should be periodic joint activities with leaders and associations. They should attempt to incorporate different groups as providers within the framework of mental health policy. International experience indicates at least three ways in which consumers become providers:

Consumers and families can be incorporated into the policy as providers.

1. Health teams: Several experiences show that consumers and families can be successfully employed in diverse services and facilities (Cohen & Natella, 1995; Goering, 1997). In developed countries, for example, they have been employed as case managers in assertive community treatment and in peer support for expanding rehabilitation services in mental health teams. This type of experience may also be replicated in developing countries, where the shortage of human resources in the field of mental health and the shortage of employment opportunities for persons with mental disorders can be eased by hiring consumers as members of mental health teams. Professionals can also benefit from the unique perspective of consumers and families on mental health. However, continuous support is required in order to prevent them from becoming overwhelmed by the stresses associated with such work.

Several experiences show that consumers and families can be employed in diverse services and facilities.

2. Community services: Their closeness to the people who face the problems of mental disorders makes it possible for consumer and family groups to run some mental health services more adequately than professionals. For example, there are promising experiences in Chile, Mexico, South Africa and Spain involving social clubs (which promote community integration of people with psychiatric disabilities), sheltered homes and various rehabilitation programmes, including vocational rehabilitation and social enterprises. Ministries of health can encourage these types of interventions, which can be effective at low cost, by establishing mechanisms for purchasing them from consumer and family groups that act as providers.

There are several instances of consumers and families running social clubs, sheltered homes and rehabilitation programmes.

3. Mental health advocacy: By participating in advocacy groups, people with mental disorders and their families not only help other individuals or communities to protect their rights but also improve their own mental health. Such participation has led to increased coping skills, self-esteem, confidence and feelings of well-being, and to expanded social networks. These are all factors of importance in relation to mental health. (See Chapter 2.7.4.) Consequently, ministries of health should make sure that the implementation of policy includes the participation of people with mental disorders and their families in advocacy groups.

Participation in advocacy groups helps consumers and families to improve mental health.

Key points: Empowerment of providers to deliver mental health interventions

- Incentives can be used with public providers to improve efficiency, quality, flexibility and responsiveness to the needs and expectations of populations.

- Contracting and regulation with private providers can help to prevent perverse incentives and encourage consistency with the objectives of mental health policy.

- Consumers and families, mutual aid groups, traditional health workers and NGOs can play a role in policy, plans and programmes whenever possible and appropriate.

- Sectors other than health can contribute towards delivering some mental health interventions.

Step 6. Reinforce intersectoral coordination

Box 12 shows examples of mental health interventions that are delivered to populations through sectors other than the health sector. (See Annex 1.) In these cases the tasks of mental health professionals in the ministry of health are as follows:

> coordinating activities with professionals from other ministries in order to formulate, implement and evaluate mental health interventions (e.g. meeting professionals of the ministry of education with a view to developing mental health promotion programmes in primary schools);

> supporting mental health professionals in health districts to implement district intersectoral interventions (e.g. meeting professionals from other sectors, such as those of housing, social services and employment in order to develop community care for people with schizophrenia);

> supporting mental health professionals in health districts in order to enhance coordination among local health teams and teams from other sectors (e.g. meeting health district teams, local social teams and mental health teams with a view to developing a programme on mother and infant bonding in poor communities).

Ministries of health sho facilitate coordination w other sectors at the nat and local levels.

Box 12. Examples of intersectoral mental health interventions*

Issue	Intervention	Sector
Promotion and prevention	Mother and infant bonding	Social services
	Prevention in the field of mental health	Social services, education, labour, justice, housing
	Promotion and prevention in the field of mental health in schools	Education
Intellectual disability	Salt or water iodization	Commerce, water supply
Suicide	Gun control	Justice
	Gas detoxification	Commerce
Schizophrenia	Community care	Housing, social services, education, employment
Alcohol and drug abuse	Culture-specific treatment	Social services, employment

* the examples are not specific recommendations for action.

Figure 2 illustrates the relationships between policy, plan, programme, interventions, supporting organization, health providers and intersectoral coordination in the field of mental health.

In order to respond to needs and demands it is necessary to prioritize promotional, preventive and therapeutic interventions, which are delivered to populations by qualified health providers. A supporting organization in ministries of health and health districts is needed in order to ensure access to these interventions. Adequate intersectoral coordination is required for the delivery of some mental health interventions by sectors outside the health sector.

Figure 2: Implementation of mental health policy, plan and programme

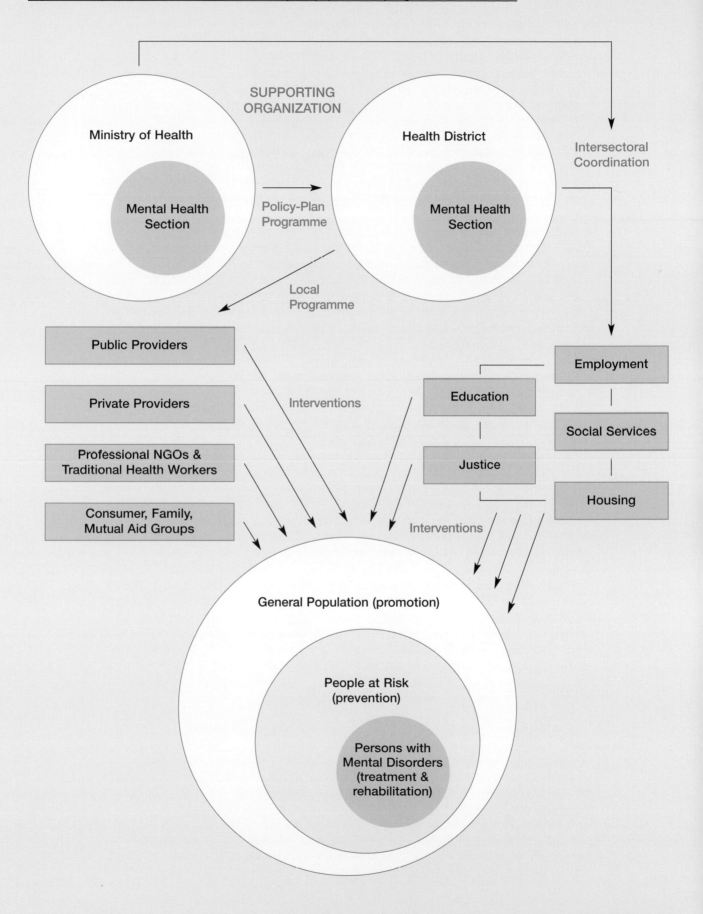

Step 7. Promote interactions among stakeholders

In order to ensure the delivery of mental health interventions that respond to the needs of a population it is necessary for multiple interactions to occur between the stakeholders. These interactions happen at different levels of the organization of a country or region.

5.7.1 Interaction between the ministry of health and other national or regional stakeholders

All the stakeholders listed in Box 2 who may have been invited to participate in the formulation of mental health policy are potential candidates for involvement in the interactions needed for implementation. At this stage, however, preference should be given to those with specific roles and responsibilities in the plans/programme concerned. For this purpose the following types of stakeholders seem to be the most relevant.

> **Stakeholders with responsibility for funding:** The mental health professionals at the ministry of health should map the mental health system in order to understand the level of current resources, the principal sources of funding and how they are used in the different service provision sectors. (See the module *Mental Health Financing*.) It is also necessary to cost the interventions that have been prioritized in the plan or programme, utilizing the activities formulated in the guidelines according to standards. (See module on *Planning and Budgeting to Deliver Services for Mental Health* for a method of costing services or programmes.)

> **Stakeholders with responsibility for provision:** Although the health districts are usually in charge of relating directly to providers, the ministry of health can facilitate this process. Interactions with national organizations can be assisted. In this case the most important goals are to obtain support for the activities proposed in the plan or programme and to overcome possible barriers.

If the mental health plan/programme includes interventions to be implemented by sectors other than health, the mental health professionals in the ministry of health should interact with their counterparts in the respective government agencies. In this case it is necessary to define how the funds of each institution are going to be managed, how they are going to be allocated to the local level and how the activities and monitoring are going to be carried out jointly or in a coordinated fashion.

> **Stakeholders with responsibility for regulation:** As described in the *Quality Improvement* module, professional associations can play a significant role in the formulation and implementation of guidelines and standards. The mental health professionals in the ministry of health can develop alliances with these organizations in order to build synergy for the plan or programme. Consumer, family and other advocacy organizations at the national or regional level can also contribute enormously towards making the plan or programme known, so that the local groups can support the delivery of interventions that are accessible and of high quality.

5.7.2 Interaction between health districts and the ministry of health

The successful implementation of a mental health policy requires a collaborative and coordinated relationship between mental health professionals at the district/local and national/regional levels. It is not unusual to encounter different visions and tensions between these levels.

One of the most important issues in this interaction is the degree of decentralization that the country or region requires in accordance with the general administrative structure, the level of development of mental health services and the social and cultural characteristics

The delivery of interven requires interactions between stakeholders at different levels of the organization of a countr or region.

The ministry of health should interact with stakeholders with responsibility for fundin provision and regulatior

One of the most importa issues in the interaction between health districts the ministry is the degre of decentralization.

72

of the population. Sometimes it is essential to have a strong vertical national or regional plan and programme in order to facilitate the development of local mental health services. In other instances an autonomous district plan or programme with no interference from central government is necessary in order to facilitate the development of innovative mental health services that respond appropriately to the particular needs of local communities.

> **District plan/programme versus national or regional plan/programme:** Each country or region should evaluate the advantages and disadvantages of developing one central mental health plan/programme, several district plans or programmes or even more decentralized plans/programmes. In any of these cases an agreement should be negotiated between health districts and the ministry of health in order to define objectives, strategies and priority interventions that are compatible between the two levels. The end result of this process should be the adoption of an explicit local plan/programme, either identical or different from that for the country or region.

> **Allocation of funds from national or regional level to district level:** As described in the *Mental Health Financing* module, funds from the national or regional level can be allocated to the district plan/programme through different mechanisms, each with pros and cons. Some examples of these mechanisms are:

- capitation, i.e. equal share of resources per head of population;
- formulae that reflect differences in the prevalence of mental disorders and risk factors (e.g. poverty, drug abuse, domestic violence);
- formulae that reflect the existing mental health resources and the cost of providing services (e.g. there will be relatively high salaries and increased transportation costs in some isolated zones);
- a protected portion of funds for the implementation of a national priority.

> **Commissioning between ministry of health and health districts:** Commissioning and contracting may be undertaken between the ministry of health and the health districts, reflecting arrangements made between managers or purchasers and providers. (See *Mental Health Financing* module and *Planning and Budgeting to Deliver Services for Mental Health* module.) In these contracts the ministry of health agrees to transfer a certain amount of funds and technical support and the health districts agree to deliver a certain amount of mental health interventions through public and/or private providers. Contracts are useful mechanisms whereby expectations can be clearly indicated in quantitative and qualitative terms. These expectations should be mutually agreed and reinforced with rewards and penalties.

5.7.3 Interaction between health districts and providers

The mental health professionals in the health districts can relate to the individuals, teams or institutions accredited for the provision of mental health services. The way in which this happens will vary according to the structure of the health system in each country or region. The relationship will also vary in accordance with the administrative organization and the roles given to the health district offices. Consequently, the functions of these mental health professionals may range from the management of mental health services in public facilities, to the purchasing and regulation of these services in the private system and coordination with other sectors delivering mental health interventions. All these functions can be conveniently utilized in order to facilitate the implementation of a mental health plan or programme.

> **Management of mental health services:** The health districts establish this type of interaction with public facilities, either implementing the plan/programme directly with control over the resources and the planning of activities, or indirectly through commissioning. In the latter arrangement a contract is drawn up with a public facility,

whereby the health district office transfers a certain amount of funds and technical support and the provider delivers a number of interventions defined in the plan/ programme in accordance with guidelines and standards.

> **Purchasing of mental health services:** As with contracts involving public facilities, health districts make contracts with private providers (for-profit or not-for-profit) in order to obtain a certain number of mental health interventions. There are different models for purchasing, such as global payment, capitation, case-rate payment and fee-for-service, and different types of contract, e.g. block contracts, cost-and-volume contracts, cost-per-service contracts and performance-based contracts. (See the module *Mental Health Financing* for details.) Depending on the existing structures and capacities in a health district, some of these mechanisms can be oriented towards expanding the mental health plan/ programme and improving efficiency, effectiveness and the quality of the interventions.

> **Regulation of mental health services:** In most developing countries there are no regulatory institutions other than the health district offices, which have to carry out various functions simultaneously. Consequently, regulation is often inadequate and the quality of services is adversely affected. The mental health professionals in the health district should spend some time on this function. By forming partnerships with consumer and family groups and with mental health workers they can help to build a culture of quality. All the health facilities that deliver interventions in accordance with the plan/programme should be accredited and should be subjected to continuous monitoring and periodic evaluations. (See the module *Quality Improvement for Mental Health*.)

> **Coordination with other sectors delivering mental health interventions:** The professionals in charge of mental health in the health district should map the principal mental health services that are provided by institutions of other sectors. (See module on *Planning and Budgeting to Deliver Services for Mental Health*.) On the basis of this information they can set priorities for concentrating efforts in a few institutions (e.g. a school programme on promotion and prevention, a workplace programme on coping with stress, pension and housing benefits for people with mental disability). In general the actions coordinated with these institutions are more productive if they have independently detected mental health problems in the people they work with or if there is an institutional commitment together with resources allocated to deal with some mental health areas.

The health district should map the principal mental health services that are provided by institutions of other sectors.

5.7.4 Interaction between consumers and providers

This is the most important level of interaction in the process of implementing the plan/programme, where the outcome of improved mental health for the people can be attained. All the previous steps should lead to a successful resolution of this interaction, with the delivery of effective interventions for promotion, prevention, treatment and rehabilitation.

The interaction between consumers and providers is the most important in the implementation of the intervention.

There are still some actions that can be carried out at this level for improving the implementation of the plan/programme. They have to do with the coordination of mental health services, support for consumer and family groups and advocacy in relation to mental health and mental disorders. Different stakeholders can be involved with these actions, depending on local realities, such as providers (e.g. primary care teams, community mental health teams), consumer or family groups with a high degree of development, social services, and professional NGOs. The professionals in charge of mental health in the health district should monitor these actions in order to ensure that they are carried out properly. They may have to facilitate the participation of stakeholders and may have to involve themselves in some activities, depending on the circumstances in the district concerned.

The health district should monitor and facilitate the participation of stakeholders. They may need to be involved in some activities, depending on the circumstances.

> Coordination of mental health services: As described in the *Organization of Services for Mental Health* module, the links between different levels of care and between the health sector and other sectors are a key issue in the matter of coordination. Regular meetings between primary care teams and secondary mental health teams should be held in order to review and improve the local referral system and to evaluate how the needs of patients are being met.

> Support for consumer and family groups: Consumer and family organizations should be empowered in order to improve the accessibility and quality of mental health services and overcome the paternalistic attitudes of some providers. (See the module *Advocacy for Mental Health* for details of how this may be achieved.)

> Advocacy for mental health and mental disorders: The stigma associated with mental disorders makes it necessary to develop an advocacy movement in order to change local cultures. There is a need for a higher awareness of the role of mental health in the quality of life and for protection of the rights of people with mental disorders. Some of the targets for advocacy activities are the general population, consumer and family groups, professional NGOs, general health workers, mental health workers, and local planners and policy-makers. (See the module *Advocacy for Mental Health* for details.)

Key points: Interacting to implement policy through plans and programmes

- The ministry of health interacts with funding agencies (ministry of finance, insurance, donor agencies), provision stakeholders (health workers, NGOs, mutual aid groups) and regulation stakeholders (professional associations, advocacy groups).

- The ministry of health should allocate funds to districts and enter into contracts in order to assure the delivery of interventions.

- Health districts should manage public services, arrange the purchasing of services from private providers, regulate all services and coordinate activities with other sectors.

- Providers should interact with consumers in order to coordinate services, support consumer and family groups and facilitate advocacy activities.

> Guinea-Bissau

At independence in 1974, Guinea-Bissau inherited a health care system that was centralized, curative and hospital-based. Within a few years a nationwide primary health care system was set up. A mental health component has been developed since 1983, with the help of an international expert. This component consisted mainly of a diagnostic phase, involving participant observation of traditional healers aimed at discovering the extent to which their functions were complementary to psychiatry, and an epidemiological investigation of people visiting basic health care facilities. The second phase involved training 850 primary care workers, their supervision every three months, and supplying basic psychotropic medication.

There were no sociocultural impediments to this public health approach. The costs of such a policy are low if a functioning primary care system exists and if buildings and salaries are already funded. In 1994 the needs of every 54 inhabitants were covered with one US dollar. The primary care workers were able to increase their recognition rates for mental disorders from 31% to 85%, and 82% of the patients received appropriate basic pharmacological treatment for major depression, psychosis and epilepsy. Patients and families were satisfied with the care received and they reported a decrease in symptoms. The activities were sustained for 10 years (De Jong, 1996).

Comments
Although no explicit policy was formulated, some elements from Chapter 2 (Developing a mental health policy: essential steps) can be recognized:

- information about the population's needs from the epidemiological investigation of people visiting primary care facilities;
- gathering evidence from participant observation of traditional health workers;
- involvement of an international expert;
- some of the areas for action, namely financial aspects, basic information system, organization of services, early treatment, essential drug procurement and human resource training.

Furthermore, some elements from Chapter 3 (Developing a mental health plan) can also be identified:

- priority-setting of major strategies, i.e. diagnostic phase, intervention in the health system (e.g. training) and intervention with people (primary care workers, with supervision every three months);
- time frame and resources;
- priority-setting of three mental and neurological problems, i.e. depression, psychosis and epilepsy.

> Pakistan

Pakistan is a large country of approximately 140 million people, of whom 72% live in rural areas. The literacy rate is about 30%. There are five psychiatric hospitals and nearly 200 psychiatrists. With the support of WHO a policy decision was made in 1986 to integrate mental health into primary care, to develop human resources so as to provide mental health care, to reduce the stigma attached to mental disorders and to develop models of community mental health care.

Successful training courses for health workers, spiritual healers and schoolteachers have been completed in some provinces, resulting in an increased understanding of mental disorders and a reduction in stigma. The 1912 Lunacy Act was replaced in 1992 by a new Mental Health Act. The number of psychiatrists increased from 120 in 1987 to 197 in 1997. A training package for primary care physicians has been developed with the aim of enabling them to recognize, manage and refer priority mental disorders. A curriculum for psychiatric nursing has been produced and postgraduate courses have been initiated. A demonstration area was established in Rawalpindi in order to evaluate community models of mental health care and it has been replicated in other areas of the country (Planning Commission, Pakistan, 1998).

Comments

The implementation of a national mental health policy in Pakistan clearly demonstrates the importance of developing the different areas for action in a comprehensive way (as described in Section 2):

- intersectoral collaboration - training of schoolteachers;
- legislation - a new Mental Health Act was approved;
- advocacy - increased understanding of mental disorders and reduction of stigma;
- research and evaluation - a demonstration area was created for the evaluation of community models;
- organization of services - integration of mental health into primary care;
- human resources - mental health training of health workers and traditional health workers, increased number of psychiatrists, training of psychiatric nurses.

> Chile

Chile has a population of 15 000 000, 85% of which is urban. The literacy rate is 95%. Although the country has had successful public health programmes for 50 years, especially in the fields of infectious diseases, birth delivery and nutrition, no mental health policy was formulated before 1990. In that year a mental health policy and plans were adopted nationally, whereby a mental health team was established in the Ministry of Health and at least one professional was placed in charge of mental health in each of the 28 health districts. The main strategies involved the integration of mental health care into primary care, the psychosocial rehabilitation of people with psychiatric disabilities, the prevention and treatment of alcohol and drug abuse and domestic violence and the treatment of victims of torture and other violations of human rights that had occurred between 1973 and 1990.

A new national plan and programme for mental health and psychiatric care were formulated in 1999 following a political crisis involving the Ministry of Health and the trade unions at the main mental hospital. The crisis, which arose because of inadequate psychiatric care for discharged patients, was resolved with a new comprehensive national plan and an increase in the mental health budget (Ministry of Health, Chile, 2000). The following changes in mental health services have taken place over a period of 12 years:

- the number of psychiatrists working in public services doubled to more than 300;
- long-stay beds decreased from 2516 to 1169;
- new services were introduced, namely 33 day hospitals, 41 community mental health teams, 60 sheltered homes serving 476 persons, and 46 social clubs;
- than 200 psychologists were incorporated into one-third of primary care facilities;
- more than 60 consumer and family groups were formed.

Comment

This example highlights two aspects of Chapter 5 (Implementation issues for policy, plans and programmes).

- *Political support*: The first national mental health policy of the country was formulated in the middle of a major change in the political context, namely the transition from dictatorship to democracy. At the time, mental health care, along with other social issues, was highly valued by the population, and the strategies prioritized responded to the people's needs in the areas of primary health care, disability, problems with alcohol and drugs, domestic violence and torture.
- *Supporting organization*: One of the crucial factors in developing mental health services and programmes in all regions of the country was the establishment of a mental health team in the Ministry of Health and of at least one professional in charge of mental health in each of the 28 health districts. These professionals coordinate the various public providers, NGOs, and consumer and family groups in local networks.

> Spain

In 1986 the General Public Health Law was passed which included a chapter on mental health. This law facilitated the transformation of psychiatric hospitals, deinstitutionalization, the mainstreaming of mental health and its development in primary care and community programmes. Mental health centres were developed for psychiatric ambulatory care, inpatient units were opened in general hospitals and therapeutic communities were created for the treatment and rehabilitation of persons with the most serious mental disorders (Montejo & Espino, 1998).

After 10 years of implementation of this psychiatric reform, large changes have occurred in some of the autonomous communities, e.g. Andalusia, Asturias and Madrid. In these regions the number of beds in psychiatric hospitals decreased from about 100 to fewer than 25 per 100 000 inhabitants. After an average stay in hospital of 21 years, people were able to return to their families in 25% of the cases, while 50% of them were able to live in sheltered accommodation. Approximately 500 mental health centres have been opened with an average coverage of 87 000 people. Ninety-five inpatient psychiatric units in general hospitals and 108 day hospitals have been created. In several regions, social services have developed rehabilitation programmes, including social enterprises with paid jobs for persons with mental disabilities. Clinical training programmes for psychiatrists and psychologists have been set up, allowing a significant increase in the numbers of these professionals.

Comment

Spain provides a good example of a country that has been able to make deep transformations in the organization of services, using mental health resources that were formerly concentrated in large psychiatric hospitals. Mental health centres, day hospitals and psychiatric units in general hospitals are coordinated in well-organized networks of services. There is also intersectoral collaboration with social services that provide housing, rehabilitation programmes and social enterprises.

Spain also demonstrates the importance of consultation and negotiation among stakeholders when policy is being developed and implemented. Although the national mental health policy was issued through the General Public Health Law, there has been variation in the pace and extent of its implementation in the different autonomous communities, depending on local political contexts and the influence of different stakeholders.

> Brazil

Brazil, the largest country in South America, has 166 million inhabitants and the world's ninth largest economy. The distribution of income is extremely unbalanced, with a large poor population and a low literacy rate. During the 1960s the Ministry of Health implemented a policy of contracting with private psychiatric hospitals in accordance with the prevailing view that persons with mental disorders should be excluded from society. This led to the development of 313 psychiatric hospitals with 85 037 beds.

As of 1982, voices were raised in denunciation of human rights violations in psychiatric hospitals. Some states began reforming mental health care by improving the treatment and conditions of persons in psychiatric hospitals and setting up psychosocial treatment centres for the community care of persons with serious mental disorders. Consumers and families became increasingly involved in the process of defining policies, along with mental health professionals. Psychiatric reform in Italy and the Declaration of Caracas also influenced policy development. An epidemiological study in three states was carried out in 1992. The national Ministry of Health introduced the following strategies in 1991:

- The financial mechanisms for mental health interventions were changed in line with the new Unified Health System.
- A Board of Mental Health State Coordinators was established to implement the new model of mental health services.
- Stakeholder participation was encouraged in 1992 when a national mental health conference was attended by over 2000 persons.
- Advice was given to parliament with a view to changing the legislation on mental health.
- International exchange was provided with support from PAHO/WHO.

These strategies led to a decrease in the number of beds in psychiatric hospitals by 30% in 10 years. In 2001 there were 52 586 such beds. During the same period there was an increase to 295 in the number of psychosocial treatment centres. Various community care initiatives have been carried out in the South-Eastern Region, which has the country's highest gross domestic product. For example, psychiatric beds in general hospitals, halfway homes, and different types of rehabilitation programmes (including social enterprises) have been implemented in several states. A new national mental health law has been approved after a 12-year parliamentary process (Alves & Valentini, 2002).

Comments
Brazil illustrates how national policy, even in a large federal country with many autonomous states, can have a significant impact on most regions: in the 1960s, institutionalization and the exclusion of persons with mental disorders were promoted, whereas in the 1990s there was a move towards community care and social integration. Interesting interactions have occurred between the federal government and the state governments. On the one hand, some states have pioneered transformations in psychiatric care and have thus influenced national policy on mental health. On the other hand, once the national policy was implemented it influenced the local policies of the different states.

The following elements of policy development and implementation are present in this example:

- *Information about the needs of the population:* The advocacy movement made evident some of the basic needs of persons in psychiatric hospitals and an epidemiological study provided information on the magnitude and characteristics of mental disorders.
- *Gathering evidence from other countries:* Lessons were gained from psychiatric reform and the development of community care in Italy. The first initiatives implemented in a few Brazilian states were developed as pilot projects.
- *Consultation and negotiation:* Consumers, families, mental health professionals and other stakeholders participated in several local and national meetings at which mental health policies were analysed.
- *Exchanges with other countries:* PAHO/WHO has played an important role in facilitating this process.
- *Supporting organization:* A Board of Mental Health State Coordinators was established.
- *Allocation of funds:* New financial mechanisms were introduced in accordance with the Unified Health System.

7. Barriers and solutions to supporting advocacy

Box 15 summarizes some of the main obstacles that mental health professionals in health ministries may face during the process of formulating and implementing new mental health policy, plans and programmes, and suggests ways in which these professionals can overcome the difficulties. More detailed explanations of some of the points in Box 15 are given subsequently.

Box 15. Suggestions for overcoming barriers to the development and implementation of mental health policy, plans and programmes*

Barriers	Solutions
1. Some stakeholders are resistant to the changes introduced by new mental health policy.	- Adopt an "all-winners approach", ensuring that the needs of all stakeholders are taken into account.
2. Health authorities do not believe in the effectiveness of mental health interventions.	- Develop pilot projects and evaluate their impact on health and consumer satisfaction. - Ask for technical reports from international experts.
3. The country is not very sensitized to mental health issues.	- Study the prevalence of mental health problems among persons using health facilities. - Make a rapid appraisal of the mental health needs of the population.
4. There is no consensus among the country's stakeholders in mental health about how to formulate and/or implement a mental health policy.	- Return to the values, principles, objectives and areas for action and ensure that most people support them. - Review what is at stake for the different leaders if the policy is implemented.
5. Insufficient resources are allocated to mental health in the ministry of health.	- Focus the implementation of the mental health policy on a demonstration area and perform cost-effectiveness studies. - Provide technical and financial support for mental health consumer and family organizations.
6. Insufficient human resources are trained in mental health care.	- Use mental health professionals to train and support general health teams to prevent and treat most common mental health problems. - Support consumer, family and mutual aid groups. - Work conjointly with traditional health workers (Ministry of Health, Botswana,1992; Freeman, 1999).

Barriers	Solutions
7. Other basic health priorities (immunization, nutrition, HIV/AIDS) compete with mental health care for funding.	- Link mental health programmes to other health priorities (e.g. reproductive health, child development), incorporating mental health interventions as a contribution to the achievement of general health goals (Freeman, 2000).
8. Primary care teams feel overburdened by their workload and refuse to accept the introduction of new mental health policy, plans and programmes.	- Listen to their needs and try to understand them. - Show them that persons with mental disorders are already a hidden part of their burden. If mental health disorders are identified and treated the burden will decrease.
9. Primary care teams do not believe in the effectiveness of mental health interventions and continue working only with physical illnesses.	- Organize periodic visits to primary care teams by mental health specialists who can demonstrate how mental health treatments operate. - Be persistent and consistent with your messages to the primary care teams.
10. Links between primary and secondary care are not working well. Access to psychiatric care is difficult and primary care teams place obstacles in the way of receiving mental health patients back.	- Reinforce the mental health supporting organization in the health districts and its role of coordinating the two levels. - Conduct frequent meetings between representatives of both teams so as to help them to reach an agreement that works well for the people.
11. There is no sector outside the health sector that seems interested in mental health. The other sectors are preoccupied with their own plans and do not see mental health as relevant to their work.	- Meet professionals from other ministries (e.g. education, social welfare, labour). - Review their priorities with them and demonstrate that persons with mental disorders are already demanding services from them. - Establish joint areas of work.
12. Many mental health specialists do not want to work either in community facilities or with primary care teams, preferring to remain in hospitals.	- Develop incentives for community care. - Obtain a fund to support research on community care. - Bring experts from other countries to act as models for community care.
13. Mental health services are overcrowded and affected by long waiting times, and consequently do not have time to work with primary care.	- Support mental health professionals in health districts so that they can help the local teams to distribute their functions and time. - Teach them to delegate work on primary care to consumer, family and mutual aid groups, as well as traditional health workers, where possible.

Barriers	Solutions
14. Trade unions in psychiatric hospitals resist changes to community care because they fear job losses.	- Offer them recycling training to community care, general health care or other available options with salary maintenance. - Do not dismiss anyone on the sole ground that a hospital is closing down.

* the examples are not specific recommendations for action.

> **Stakeholders resistant:** In any social process that produces changes in the structure of a particular society, especially in relation to the power structure, there are people who feel threatened because they anticipate losses in power, money or other areas. The process of transforming psychiatric hospitals is a classic case, where psychiatrists and staff on the one hand and patients and families on the other feel that they may lose something (e.g. time for research, meals during working time, a safe place to hide, a peaceful home).

In order to guard against this threat it is necessary for the principal stakeholders to become convinced that the new policy will bring benefits to all of them. The mental health professionals in the ministry of health should actively listen to expressions of needs by stakeholders and should try to negotiate agreements that could increase support for the policy. It is also necessary to avoid hidden agendas, e.g. using the new policy as a pretext for dismissing staff. In general, stakeholders will be more satisfied with their work or with the services that they receive when a new mental health policy of the kind described in this module is introduced.

> **Health authorities not committed to mental health:** Health authorities, like most of the general population, do not have much knowledge of mental disorders and harbour numerous myths about them. One of the most troublesome misconceptions is that mental health interventions are ineffective and that, consequently, funding allocated to them will not benefit the population.

Some strategies for sensitizing health authorities are described in the *Advocacy for Mental Health module*. Moreover, the mental health professionals in the ministry of health can devote part of their time to supporting pilot projects in some health districts where mental health outcomes and consumer satisfaction can be evaluated in the short term. The authorities can be invited to visit the projects and presented with the results. A technical report based on the visits of international experts, as described in Chapter 2.4 of this module, can contribute to this process.

> **Population not sensitized to mental health:** Countries pass through diverse historical processes. In some periods there may be many matters other than mental health which hold people's attention, interest and motivation. There are times when the visibility of mental health issues declines.

In this situation the mental health professionals in the ministry of health may decide to carry out a study on the magnitude and importance of the problem. As described in Chapter 2.1 of this module, formal research or rapid appraisal can be conducted in accordance with the available resources and technical capacities.

> **Lack of agreement among mental health stakeholders:** In some countries, mental health professionals in the ministry of health may obtain political support from the minister to formulate or implement mental health policy. However, some well-known mental

health leaders in the country may argue against the proposed policy and they may gather support among other stakeholders.

As noted in Chapter 2.3 (Consultation and negotiation) of this module it is important to reach basic agreements among stakeholders on the vision, values, principles, objectives and areas for action of the policy. It may also be necessary for mental health professionals in the ministry of health to hold discussions with leaders opposed to the policy. This will help to develop an understanding of what is at stake for these leaders if the policy is implemented.

> **Insufficient resources for mental health:** This is most frequently the case in developing countries.

The mental health professionals in the ministry of health can confront this obstacle by focusing scarce resources in a demonstration area (see Chapter 5.4) where the vision and main strategies of the mental health policy can be implemented and evaluated. It is important to conduct cost-effectiveness studies in this area and to use the results as a means of convincing decision-makers to invest in mental health. Another option is to utilize some resources for supporting consumer and other advocacy groups (see the module *Advocacy for Mental Health*) so that they can reach a higher level of development and persuade the national authorities to allocate more resources to the mental health policy.

> **Insufficient human resources trained in mental health:** This can be a serious limitation in developing countries, especially those with particularly low incomes, whose psychiatrists, for instance, have to be trained in developed countries. Many of them do not return because they take advantage of the professional opportunities available in developed countries.

There are various ways in which the mental health professionals in the ministry of health can face this difficulty. First, central funding can be allocated to health districts for the training of primary care teams on the prevention and treatment of the most common mental disorders and for the enhancement of links between primary and secondary care.

Second, support in the form of funds and technical capacities can be transferred to consumer and mutual aid groups in order to empower them, facilitate the development of the advocacy movement and reinforce social networks. (See the module *Advocacy for Mental Health*.) These measures have all been demonstrated to decrease the utilization of mental health services.

Third, in many countries traditional health workers offer an excellent means of multiplying the number of health staff. Properly trained, they can learn to differentiate mild emotional problems that they can treat effectively from serious mental disorders that require treatment in health facilities.

Fourth, conditions can be attached to the granting of funds for overseas study. For example, trainees can be obliged to return to their country of origin in order to serve for a minimum period once their overseas training has been completed.

> **Other health priorities compete with mental health:** Many health priorities compete for resources with mental health. Immunization campaigns, nutritional supplementation and the prevention of HIV/AIDS, for instance, are frequently given a higher priority than mental disorders.

In these cases the proposed strategy is to link mental health plans or programmes with other health priorities in a way that makes mental health interventions acceptable as a means of helping to achieve general health goals (Freeman, 2000).

> **Primary health care teams resistant:** As a rule the members of these teams are already overburdened with general health activities and they often perceive mental health programmes as an additional workload. This is especially true where the training of health technicians and professionals does not include sufficient attention to mental health skills.

Professionals in ministries of health or health districts should spend time interacting with primary care teams in order to learn about their needs, their reasons for being resistant and their motivations. An incentive that can encourage primary care technicians and professionals to incorporate mental health into their daily work is the receipt of continuous training on the subject. This favours career development and the improvement of the quality of service on a continuing basis.

> **Primary health care teams doubtful about effectiveness of mental health interventions:** Primary care teams usually harbour the same misconceptions about mental disorders as the general population. They are not aware of the effectiveness of pharmacological and psychosocial interventions.

The strategy that has proved effective for introducing mental health to primary care has been to set aside time for regular contact between primary care workers and mental health specialists. One way of doing this is for a psychiatrist, psychologist or any other mental health worker to visit a primary care facility periodically, i.e. once or twice a month. During the visits, promotional and preventive activities are performed together, persons with mental disorders are assessed and treated conjointly, theories and clinical cases are discussed, referral and counter-referral procedures are agreed, and administrative issues are resolved.

> **Insufficient linking between primary and specialist care:** Overburdened primary care teams sometimes refer all persons with mental disorders to the specialist level. They do not attempt to treat persons with mild disorders or to carry out promotional or preventive interventions. This overburdens the mental health specialists, and long waiting times and/or obstacles arise which make it very difficult for the required treatments to be given. Furthermore, persons who receive psychiatric treatment are often not referred back to primary care, and this adds to the burden for the specialists.

Mental health professionals in ministries of health should strengthen the mental health supporting organization in health districts so that they can coordinate the activities of the primary and specialist care levels. This requires frequent meetings with representatives of both levels. They should reach basic agreements about referral and counter-referral procedures. Mental health policy, plans and programmes can help to overcome this barrier if they make the functions of both levels and the mechanisms for linking them explicit.

> **Sectors other than the health sector not interested in mental health:** It is not unusual for other sectors to set different priorities and not to visualize mental health as relevant to their work. The situation is exacerbated by insufficient knowledge and the stigma associated with mental disorders which occurs in most societies.

Professionals in ministries of health and health districts should frequently meet professionals from other ministries. It seems important to know their priorities and to find common ground on mental health policy. It is likely that persons with mental disorders are already demanding services from them or that services promoting mental health or the prevention of mental disorders are already being delivered.

Ministries of health should define areas of interest in mental health which they share with other ministries. The same process should be replicated at the health district level.

> **Mental health specialists not committed to community model:** Many psychiatrists, clinical psychologists and other mental health workers have been trained to work in hospitals, most frequently in mental hospitals. They generally have a partial view of the process, and adopt a disease model restricted to the most severe mental disorders during episodes involving the most serious symptoms. These professionals are also offered incentives to work in hospitals, e.g. higher salaries, opportunities for research, further training and academic careers. It is not rare that the majority of them prefer to continue working in hospitals.

Professionals in ministries of health and health districts should consider introducing incentives for mental health professionals working in community facilities and supporting primary care teams. Incentives may be monetary or related to career advancement. It is also important to have funds for supporting research on community care, which can make this practice more attractive.

If there is no experience of community care in the country or region concerned the ministry of health can consider the following alternatives:

- bringing experts in community care from other regions or countries;
- developing pilot projects and/or demonstration areas in community care, which can be used as training centres for this type of practice;
- sending mental health professionals to other regions or countries for training in community care.

> **Mental health services overcrowded:** This is usually the case in developing countries, where the numbers of mental health specialists are insufficient for the needs of the populations. Psychiatrists and psychologists have to care for too many people and do not have time to work in conjunction with primary care teams.

Health districts can help mental health teams to improve the organization of their functions and time. These teams should delegate part of their work to primary care teams, to consumer, family and mutual aid groups, and to traditional health workers and other resources that may be available. In this way the mental health teams can find time to link with primary care teams and help them to increase their capacity. The mental health teams should be informed that this strategy can improve access, quality and people's satisfaction with care.

> **Labour unions at psychiatric hospitals resistant:** This has been a frequent obstacle to psychiatric reform in several countries. When community care is implemented, hospital workers fear the loss of jobs or privileges. The threat is greater if the number of beds is reduced or the hospital closes down. Ideological positions adopted against institutionalization can also contribute to this situation if blame is placed on the hospital workers.

Professionals in health ministries should guarantee that no hospital worker will lose employment or salary because of the implementation of mental health policies. As the process of deinstitutionalization continues and community facilities are provided the workers should be offered training in community care skills. Several examples exist of mental health workers in hospitals who have become excellent community workers. As this does not always happen, however, provision should be made for moving some to other positions in the health system.

8. Recommendations and conclusions

Developing and implementing mental health policy, plans and programmes in a country or region is a complex process. Many factors have to be considered and the needs of various stakeholders have to be taken into consideration.

In this module, policy-makers and public health professionals can find a method for organizing actions at different stages and for facing challenges and barriers. Inevitably, most of the solutions will not be found in the module but in the realities of local communities. It is hoped that the information given will help to lighten the required tasks and provide guidance in decision-making.

The professionals in charge of policy, plans and programmes will have to develop skills in the areas of epidemiology, management, planning, budgeting, negotiation and lobbying. The process requires moving between theory and practice, while interacting with real people and their circumstances.

The specific circumstances of developing and implementing mental health policy, plans and programmes can vary enormously from one country to another. The steps for developing policy, plans and programmes in this module have to be adapted to the particular conditions of the countries concerned.

Although there is variation between countries it is essential that countries develop policy, plans and programmes for mental health. Equipped with a policy, plan and programmes, a country is well placed to systematically improve the mental health of its population.

Implementing the steps in this module may be a slow process requiring the mobilization of political will. It may take five to ten years before outcomes are achieved in the population. Nevertheless, the experiences of several countries or regions show that these steps are feasible for the development and implementation of mental health policies, plans and programmes. The whole process can produce positive mental health outcomes and the population of a country or region can receive the following benefits (WHO, 2001a):

- alleviation of symptoms associated with mental disorders;
- improved functioning in various areas (e.g. family, social, education, work);
- enhancement of productivity at work;
- improvement in the quality of life of persons with mental disorders and their families;
- prevention of psychological and social disability;
- reduction in mortality (e.g. suicide).

People with different needs are the focus of mental health promotion, the prevention of disorders, and treatment and rehabilitation. Notwithstanding the complexity of the process and the many obstacles presented, improvements in the mental health, well-being, functioning and quality of life of people with mental disorders provide more than adequate motivation for the development and implementation of mental health policies, plans and programmes.

Developing and implementing of mental health policy, plans and programmes in a country or region is a complex process.

The professionals in charge of policy, plans and programmes will have to develop several skills.

Equipped with a policy, plan and programmes, a country is well placed to systematically improve the mental health of its population.

Annex 1. Examples of effective mental health interventions

Box 16. Examples of effective mental health interventions*

Promotion and prevention	Developing mother and infant bonding in poor communities (Driscoll, 1998; Freeman, 2000)
	Non-specific prevention in the field of mental health: combating child abuse, abandonment of elderly people and trauma in migrants and refugees (Tansella, 2000)
	Mental health promotion in schools (Freeman, 2000)
	Developing coping skills and good peer relationships among schoolchildren (Driscoll, 1998)
Intellectual disability	Use of iodine by prospective mothers in areas at risk (salt iodization, water iodization or use of iodized oil and Lugol's solution) (WHO, 1998b, 2001a)
	Screening of alcohol problems in pregnant women, supportive counselling and early treatment (WHO, 1998b, 2001a)
	Screening of all neonates for phenylketonuria and treatment with low-phenylalanine diet (WHO, 1998b, 2001a)
Epilepsy	Adequate prenatal care, safe delivery, control of fever in children, prevention of brain injury and control of parasitic and infectious diseases (WHO, 1998b, 2001a)
Depression	Outpatient treatment in primary care (WHO, 1998c, 2001a)
Suicide	Early recognition and treatment of people with depression
	Gun control, gas detoxification, control of toxic substances, physical barriers to deter jumping from high places (WHO, 1998b, 2001a)
Schizophrenia	Community care: outpatient care, day centres, supported employment, support for families, supported housing, community mental health teams (Lesage & Tansella, 1993; Knapp, Chisholm, Astin et al., 1997; WHO, 2001a)
	Acute day hospital care is an alternative to inpatient admission for selected patients (Department of Health, UK, 1996;)
	Prescribing certain antipsychotics, such as clozapine, offsets the costs of inpatient care (Department of Health, UK, 1996)
Alcohol and drug abuse	Brief intervention for persons with early drinking problems by primary care professionals (WHO, 2001a)
	Counselling, behavioural therapies and self-help groups for alcohol and drug dependence (WHO, 2001a)

* the examples are not specific recommendations for action.

The examples given in Box 16 are described in more detail below.

Promotion and prevention

> *Developing mother and infant bonding in poor communities:* Intensive interventions involving home visits for several years, parent support, training in relationship skills, advice on community resources and help in relation to the educational and occupational goals of parents. There is evidence of improved cognitive development of babies, fewer behavioural problems during adolescence and a lower risk of depression.

> *Non-specific prevention:* Combating child abuse, abandonment of elderly people and trauma in migrants and refugees; multisectoral interventions aimed at combating poverty, domestic isolation, powerlessness (resulting, for example, from low educational levels and economic dependence) and the oppression of women.

> *Mental health promotion in schools:* Interventions delivered by trained teachers at both the primary and secondary school levels include life skills for the prevention of HIV/AIDS, the prevention of substance abuse, the promotion of mental health and the prevention of violence.

> *Developing coping skills and good peer relationships among schoolchildren:* Interventions performed in schools with either all the children or only high-risk groups, including enhancement of cognitive development, training in social skills and skills for coping with negative feelings, the development of positive attitudes towards school, controlling anger and understanding feelings. There is evidence for improved cognitive competence, less peer rejection, less shyness and more social competencies.

Intellectual disability

> *Use of iodine by prospective mothers* in areas at risk (salt iodization, water iodization or use of iodized oil and Lugol's solution: Intersectoral interventions consisting of the addition of iodine to either salt used at home or drinking-water. Alternatively, health workers can give Lugol's solution orally or iodized oil intramuscularly or orally to women at risk. There is evidence of full protection of the developing fetus during the first trimester if iodine is administered before pregnancy. Salt iodization is the most cost-effective method.

> *Screening of alcohol problems in pregnant women, supportive counselling and early treatment:* Interventions are delivered as part of medical care during pregnancy. They include a brief questionnaire administered for screening purposes to all pregnant women, counselling for those with mild or moderate alcohol-related problems (aiming for abstinence or a substantial reduction in alcohol consumption), and referral to specialized treatment if there are serious problems. There is evidence of a decrease in the abuse of alcohol in pregnant women and of a decreased incidence of fetal alcohol syndrome.

> *Screening all neonates for phenylketonuria and treatment with low-phenylalanine diet:* Interventions include blood sampling in order to determine the phenylalanine level when infants are under 7 days of age. For those with phenylketonuria a special diet is given by the time they are 3 weeks old. The parents are appropriately counselled. There is evidence of the prevention of brain damage and of a reduction in mental impairment.

Epilepsy

> *Adequate prenatal care, safe delivery, control of fever in children, prevention of brain injury and control of parasitic and infectious diseases:* Interventions among

pregnant women in primary care facilities and improvement in the quality of birth attendance during delivery. With regard to children, antipyretic drugs or cool baths, immunizations and environmental sanitation are provided. There is evidence of a reduction in the prevalence of epilepsy.

Depression

> *Outpatient treatment for depression in primary care:* Interventions are delivered to adolescents and adults who demand services from primary care facilities. These include the early identification of depressive symptoms, the treatment of mild and moderate disorders with antidepressant medication and individual and group psychosocial therapies, and the referral of cases of serious depression to specialists. There is evidence of decreased utilization of health services and symptomatic relief.

Suicide

> *Early recognition and treatment of people with depression:* Interventions are provided by psychiatric or community mental health teams for persons with mental disorders associated with an elevated risk of suicide (depression, alcohol and drug abuse, and schizophrenia), including ambulatory, day hospital and inpatient care. There is evidence of a reduction in suicide rates in persons with depression as a consequence of early recognition and maintenance treatment.

> *Gun control, gas detoxification, control of toxic substances, physical barriers to deter jumping from high places:* Interventions are aimed at decreasing access to instruments of suicide. They include legislation restricting the sale of handguns, the detoxification of domestic gas, a reduction in the carbon monoxide content of car emissions, limitations on the availability of toxic substances and the use of fencing on high buildings and bridges. There is evidence of a decrease in the suicide rate associated with gas detoxification and the control of car emissions.

Schizophrenia

> *Community care:* Outpatient care, day centres, supported employment, support and training for families, supported housing, and community mental health teams are involved. The interventions delivered to persons with schizophrenia and their families include psychosocial and psychopharmacological treatments. The interventions delivered to the community at large in order to reduce stigma and discrimination include public education. There is evidence for symptomatic relief, improvement in the quality of life and social integration.

> *Acute day hospital care:* This is an alternative to inpatient admission for selected patients. Interventions which are delivered during the daytime by a specialized team, to people with acute episodes of schizophrenia, include intensive psychosocial and psychopharmacological treatments. There is evidence that such interventions are as effective and less expensive than inpatient treatments.

> Prescribing certain *antipsychotics*, such as clozapine, in community settings is a cost-effective way of offsetting the costs of inpatient care. Psychiatrists may deliver both traditional and atypical antipsychotics. There is evidence of improved clinical responses, increased social integration and reduced hospitalization times with atypical antipsychotics in people giving poor responses to the traditional agents.

Alcohol and drug abuse

> *Brief interventions for persons with early drinking problems by primary care professionals:* These interventions consist of a few instructional and motivational sessions focusing on the specific behaviour of alcohol consumption, together with feedback and practical advice. There is evidence of a reduction in alcohol consumption and heavy drinking. It has also been shown that these interventions are cost-effective.

> *Counselling, behavioural therapies and self-help groups for alcohol and drug dependence:* It is recommended that the care of persons who abuse alcohol or drugs, and of their families, be shared by general practitioners and specialists. Interventions include detoxification, motivation, training in coping and problem-solving skills, and the prevention of relapses. Self-help groups also deliver interventions, as well as providing therapeutic communities and other culturally appropriate treatments. There is evidence of a cost-effective reduction in drug use and of positive consequences for health and social matters, e.g. reduced HIV infection and criminal activity.

Box 17. Principles for the development of mental health guidelines
(adapted from New Zealand Guidelines Group, 2001)

1. Guidelines should be focused on improved consumer outcomes: If possible, guidelines should target positive changes that are valued by consumers in the mental health of individuals, groups of people or populations (e.g. quality of life, functional level).

2. Guidelines should be based on the best available evidence: Apart from quantitative research and systematic reviews, data should also be obtained from well-designed qualitative studies. However, as both types of mental health research are uncommon in developing countries, other methods should be considered, e.g. agreement among a group of experts and the adaptation of guidelines developed by other regions or countries.

3. The process of guideline development should be multidisciplinary and should involve consumers: If guidelines are to be relevant the people who are expected to use and benefit from them should play a part in their development. These people are general health workers, mental health workers, representatives of relevant consumer and family groups, public health specialists and representatives of professional groups. Their involvement will improve acceptance and compliance with the guidelines.

4. Guidelines should be flexible and adaptable to different circumstances: They should consider differences in populations, geographical settings, resource availability, and consumer expectations, values and preferences. In this connection, national guidelines should be adapted to regional and local realities.

5. Guidelines should be developed in accordance with constraints on resources: If possible an economic appraisal should be included in guidelines, especially where cost data may be helpful for choosing between treatment options and influencing managerial or purchasing decisions.

6. Guidelines should be reviewed and updated regularly: They should be reviewed after an appropriate period, usually three to five years, and when new evidence becomes available.

Annex 3. Supporting the development of mental health policy, plans and programmes: functions of some key stakeholders

The functions listed here should be informed by the mental health policy and the strategies of the plan, as well as by any programmes that are adopted.

1. Functions of mental health professionals at the level of the ministry of health
- To sensitize the general population and decision-makers about mental health needs and demands and the strategies required to meet them.

- To formulate, manage, monitor and evaluate mental health legislation, policy, plans and programmes.

- To propose and implement national mental health actions in conjunction with other sectors and national organizations of consumers and families.

- To facilitate the training of health workers at both the undergraduate and graduate levels.

- To promote mental health policy evaluation and research, defining priorities and facilitating the development of research centres.

- To elaborate and implement strategies for enhancing the development and accreditation of mental health providers.

- To elaborate and distribute clinical and administrative guidelines and standards, and to facilitate processes for improving their utilization by health teams.

- To maintain a mental health information system and surveillance of the mental health of the population.

- To support the work of mental health professionals in health districts.

2. Functions of mental health professionals at the level of the health district
- To sensitize the district population and decision-makers about mental health needs and demands and the strategies to meet them.

- To formulate, manage, monitor and evaluate the district plan and programme.

- To propose and implement mental health actions in conjunction with other sectors and with district organizations of people with mental disorders and their families.

- To facilitate in-service training of general health workers and mental health workers.

- To elaborate and implement strategies for enhancing the development and accreditation of mental health providers.

- To elaborate and distribute clinical and administrative guidelines and standards and to facilitate processes for improving their utilization by health teams.

- To maintain a mental health information system and surveillance of the mental health state of the population.

- To coordinate the district mental health network through the definition of common procedures, the implementation of referral and counter-referral systems, and regular meetings with general health teams and mental health teams.

3. Functions of the coordinator of a community mental health team

- To coordinate the activities of the members of the community mental health team, in order to distribute responsibilities and ensure the accessibility, quality and continuity of interventions.

- To define procedures of referral and counter-referral with primary care teams and other mental health facilities.

- To coordinate a system of regular mental health consultations with the primary care teams of the area concerned.

- To support and coordinate activities involving people with mental disorders, their families, and mutual aid and mental health advocacy groups that work in the team's area.

- To plan and implement mental health activities in conjunction with other sectors working in the same area.

- To ensure the utilization of administrative, promotional, preventive and clinical guidelines in the regular work of the members of the team.

- To keep the records of activities and patients up-to-date and to evaluate the work of the team on a regular basis.

- To periodically assess the mental health needs and expectations of and proposals from the area's population.

4. Functions of the mental health coordinator of a primary care team

- To coordinate the mental health activities of the members of the primary care team in order to facilitate promotional and preventive interventions, early detection of mental health problems, and interventions concerned with treatment or rehabilitation.

- To define and keep current the procedures of referral and counter-referral with the community mental health team and other mental health facilities.

- To coordinate the system of regular mental health consultations by the community mental health team.

- To support and coordinate work with people who have mental disorders, their families, and mutual aid and mental health advocacy groups in the team's area.

- To plan and implement mental health actions in conjunction with other sectors working in the same area.

- To ensure the utilization of administrative, promotional, preventive and clinical guidelines in the regular work of the members of the team.

- To maintain the registration of mental health activities up-to-date and to evaluate the work of the team on a regular basis.

- To periodically assess the mental health needs, expectations and proposals of the area's population.

Mental health policy / An organized set of values, principles, objectives and areas for action to improve the mental health of a population.

Mental health plan / A detailed preformulated scheme for implementing strategies for the promotion of mental health, the prevention of mental disorders, and treatment and rehabilitation.

Mental health programme / A targeted intervention, usually short-term, with a highly focused objective for the promotion of mental health, the prevention of mental disorders, and treatment and rehabilitation.

Health district / A geographical or political division of a country, established with a view to decentralizing the functions of the ministry of health.

Mental health stakeholders / Persons and organizations with some interest in improving the mental health of a population. They include people with mental disorders, family members, professionals, policy-makers, funders and other interested parties.

Value / A cultural belief concerning a desirable mode of behaviour or end-state which guides attitudes, judgements and comparisons.

Principle / A fundamental truth or doctrine on which rules of conduct are based.

Areas for action / Complementary aspects of a policy that are separated for the purpose of planning.

Strategy / An orderly organization of activities for achieving an objective or goal.

Mental health intervention / An activity whose purpose is to promote mental health, prevent mental disorders, provide treatment or favour rehabilitation.

Provider / An organization, mental health team or institution that delivers mental health interventions to a population.

Further reading

1. Commonwealth Department of Health and Family Services, Australia (1997) *Evaluation of the National Mental Health Strategy*. Canberra: Commonwealth Department of Health and Family Services, Mental Health Branch. Australia. www.health.gov.au

2. De Jong JTV (1996) A comprehensive public mental health programme in Guinea-Bissau: a useful model for African, Asian and Latin-American countries. *Psychological Medicine*, 26:97-108.

3. Desjarlais R et al. (1995) *World mental health: problems and priorities in low-income countries*. New York: Oxford University Press Inc.

4. Driscoll L (1998) *Mental health promotion, a policy framework*. Ottawa: Policy Research International Inc.

5. Goering P et al. (1997) *Review of the best practices in mental health reform*. Ottawa: Health Canada.

6. Ministry of Health, Mental Health Unit (2000) *Plan Nacional de Salud Mental y Psiquiatria [National Mental Health and Psychiatry Plan]*. Ministry of Health, Mental Health Unit, Santiago, Chile In Spanish.

7. Planning Commission, Pakistan (1998) *Report of the Subcommittee on Mental Health and Substance Abuse for the Ninth Five Year Plan*. Planning Commission. Islamabad: Government of Pakistan.

8. Thornicroft G, Tansella M (1999) *The mental health matrix. A manual to improve services*. London: Cambridge University Press.

9. World Health Organization (1996) *Public mental health: guidelines for the elaboration and management of national mental health programmes*. Geneva: World Health Organization, Division of Mental Health and Prevention of Substance Abuse.

10. World Health Organization (1998) *Supporting governments and policy-makers*. Geneva: World Health Organization, Division of Mental Health and Prevention of Substance Abuse.

11. World Health Organization (1998) *Primary prevention of mental, neurological and psychosocial disorders*. Geneva: World Health Organization.

12. World Health Organization (1999) *Setting the WHO agenda for mental health*. Geneva: World Health Organization, Department of Mental Health and Social Change.

13. World Health Organization (2001a) Mental health: new understanding, new hope. *World Health Report 2001*. Geneva: World Health Organization.

References

1. Alarcon RD, Aguilar-Gaxiola SA (2000) Mental health policy developments in Latin America. *Bulletin of the World Health Organization*, 78(4):483-90.

2. Alves DN, Valentini W (2002) Mental health policy in Brazil. In: Hazelton M, Morral P, eds. *Mental Health: Global Perspectives and Human Rights*. London: Whurr Ed. 2003.

3. Arjonilla S, Parada IM, Pelcastre B (2000) Cuando la salud mental se convierte en una prioridad. [When mental health becomes a priority]. *Salud Mental*, 23(5):35-40. In Spanish.

4. Asioli E (2000) *Cultura y estructura para hacerse cargo del paciente en el Departamento de Salud Mental (Culture and structure to be in charge of the patient in the mental health department)*. In: *La Promoción de la Salud Mental* (Promotion of Mental Health), De Plato G & Venturini E. Bologna: Regione Emilia Romagna Press. In Spanish.

5. Barrientos G (2000) *National Mental Health Policy in Cuba*. Personal communication.

6. Bertolote JM (1992) *Planificación y administración de acciones de salud mental. [Planning and administration of mental health activities]* In: Temas de salud mental en la communidad [Topics of mental health in the community]. Washington, OPS/OMS. In Spanish.

7. Cohen H, Natella G (1995) *Trabjar en salud mental, la desmanicomialización en Rio Negro [Working on mental health, the deinstitutionalization in Rio Negro].* Buenos Aires: Lugar Editorial. In Spanish.

8. Commonwealth Department of Health and Family Services, Australia (1997) *Evaluation of the National Mental Health Strategy.* Canberra: Commonwealth Department of Health and Family Services, Mental Health Branch. www.health.gov.au

9. De Jong JTV (1996) A comprehensive public mental health programme in Guinea-Bissau: a useful model for African, Asian and Latin-American countries. *Psychological Medicine*, 26:97-108.

10. Department of Health of South Africa (1997) *White paper for the transformation of the health system in South Africa.* Pretoria: Government Gazette.

11. Department of Health of the United Kingdom (1996) *The spectrum of care: local services for people with mental health problems.* London: Department of Health.

12. Department of Health of the United Kingdom (1999) *Mental health: national service frameworks.* www.doh.gov.uk

13. Driscoll L (1998) *Mental health promotion, a policy framework.* Ottawa: Policy Research International Inc.

14. Freeman M (1999) *National health policy guidelines for improved mental health In South Africa.* (Draft document.)

15. Freeman M (2000) Using all opportunities for improving mental health - examples from South Africa. *Bulletin of the World Health Organization*, 78(4):508-10.

16. Goering P et al. (1997) *Review of the best practices in mental health reform.* Ottawa: Health Canada.

17. Goldberg D, Gournay K (1997) *The general practitioner, the psychiatrist and the burden of mental health care.* London: The Maudsley.

18. Health Canada (1998) *Review of best practices in mental health reform.* Ottawa: Clarke Institute of Psychiatry and Health Canada.

19. Kemp DR (1994) An overview of mental health policy from an international perspective. In: Kemp DR (ed). *International handbook on mental health policy.* London: Greenwood Press.

20. Knapp M et al. (1997) The cost consequences of changing the hospital-community balance: the mental health residential care study. *Psychological Medicine*, 27:681-92.

21. Lesage AD, Tansella M (1993) Comprehensive community care without long stay beds in mental hospitals: trends from an Italian good practice area. *Canadian Journal of Psychiatry*, 38:187-94.

22. Mental Health Division, Alberta Health, Canada (1993) *Working in partnership: building a better future for mental health.* Edmonton: Mental Health Division, Alberta Health, Canada.

23. Ministry of Health, Botswana (1992) *Mental health programme: action plan.* Gaborone: Ministry of Health.

24. Ministry of Health, Mental Health Unit, Chile (2000) *Plan Nacional de Salud Mental y Psiquiatria [National Mental Health and Psychiatry Plan].* Santiago: Ministry of Health, Mental Health Unit, Chile. In Spanish.

25. Ministry of Supply and Services, Canada (1988) *Mental health for Canadians: striking a balance.* Ottawa: Ministry of Supply and Services, Canada.

26. Montejo J, Espino A (1998) *Sobre los resultados de la reforma psiquiatríca y de la salud mental en España [Results of psychiatric and mental health reform in Spain].* In: García J, Espino A, Lara L (eds). La Psiquiatría en la España de Fin de Siglo *[Psychiatry in Spain at the end of the century].* Madrid: Diaz de Santos. p. 363-87. In Spanish.

27. New Zealand Guidelines Group (2001) *Evidence-based clinical practice guidelines.* Wellington: New Zealand Guidelines Group.

28. Planning Commission, Pakistan (1998) *Report of the Subcommittee on Mental Health and Substance Abuse for the Ninth Five Year Plan.* Islamabad: Government of Pakistan.

29. Pearson V (1992) Community and culture: a Chinese model of community care for the mentally ill. *International Journal of Social Psychiatry*, 38(3):163-78.

30. Phillips MR (2000) Mental health services in China (editorial). *Epidemiologia e Psichiatria Sociale*, 9(2):84-8.

31. Tansella M (2000) Making mental health services work at the primary level. *Bulletin of the World Health Organization*, 78(4):501-2.

32. Thornicroft G, Tansella M (1999) *The mental health matrix. A manual to improve services.* London: Cambridge University Press.

33. Ustun TB, Sartorius N (1995) the Background and Rationale of the WHO Collaborative Study on Psychological Problems in General Health Care.In *Mental illness in general health care: an international study.* John Wiley & Sons Ltd, West Sussex, UK.

34. World Health Organization (1984) *Mental health care in developing countries: a critical appraisal of research findings.* Geneva: World Health Organization (Technical Report Series, No. 698).

35. World Health Organization (1987) *Care for the mentally ill. Components of mental policies governing the provision of psychiatric services.* Montreal: WHO Collaborating Centre for Research and Training in Mental Health.

36. World Health Organization (1989) *Consumer Involvement in Mental Health and Rehabilitation Services.* Geneva: World Health Organization, Division of Mental Health.

37. World Health Organization (1993a) *Essential treatments in psychiatry.* Geneva: World Health Organization, Division of Mental Health.

38. World Health Organization (1993b) *Essential drugs in psychiatry.* Geneva: World Health Organization, Division of Mental Health.

39. World Health Organization (1994) *Quality assurance in mental health care: check lists and glossaries*. Geneva: World Health Organization, Division of Mental Health.

40. World Health Organization (1996) Public mental health: guidelines for the elaboration and management of national mental health programmes. Geneva: World Health Organization, Division of Mental Health and Prevention of Substance Abuse.

41. World Health Organization (1997) *An overview of a strategy to improve mental health of underserved populations*. Geneva: World Health Organization, Division of Mental Health and Prevention of Substance Abuse.

42. World Health Organization (1998a) *Supporting governments and policy-makers*. Geneva: World Health Organization, Division of Mental Health and Prevention of Substance Abuse.

43. World Health Organization (1998b) *Primary prevention of mental, neurological and psychosocial disorders*. Geneva: World Health Organization.

44. World Health Organization (1998c) *Mental Disorders in Primary Care*. Geneva: World Health Organization, Department of Mental Health and Substance Abuse.

45. World Health Organization (1999) *Setting the WHO agenda for mental health*. Geneva: World Health Organization, Department of Mental Health, Social Change and Mental Health.

46. World Health Organization (2000a) *World Health Report 2000. Health systems: improving performance*. Geneva: World Health Organization.

47. World Health Organization (2000b) *Mental health and work: impact, issues and good practices*. Geneva: World Health Organization, Department of Mental Health and Substance Abuse.

48. World Health Organization (2001a) *World Health Report 2001. Mental health: new understanding, new hope*. Geneva: World Health Organization.

49. World Health Organization (2001b) *Atlas: Mental health resources in the world 2001*. Geneva: World Health Organization, Department of Mental Health and Substance Dependence.